PRAISE FOR DR. PLATT

"Dr. Platt is an expert and renowned for his work with natural hormone replacement to enhance wellness. The findings in this thoroughly reader-friendly book are presented skillfully and clearly, making the information thoroughly accessible for the general reader. This book can substantially aid men and women, with the help of their physicians, to seek effective hormonal solutions to health conditions considered insoluble."

— MIDWEST BOOK REVIEW

"Make no mistake—this is NOT a book just for menopausal women. Men, women, and children with a myriad of chronic conditions and debilitating illnesses will finally find answers in their quest to just feel better."

— ELLEN PARRIS, *reviewer,* Palm Springs Life

"As a practicing orthopedic surgeon in Jakarta, Indonesia, with immense interest in preventive medicine, I strongly recommend this book, as it is a fantastic one, the only kind of book that prompted me to fly from the other side of the globe to meet the author in person."

— HENRY SUHENDRA, M.D., F.IC.S.

"I'm very proud, and at the same time relieved, that we have doctors like Dr. Platt, truly interested in patients' complaints and devoted to preventive medicine."

— DR. LUIS CESAR ANZOATEGUI, *professor and physician, Mato Grosso do Sul, Brazil*

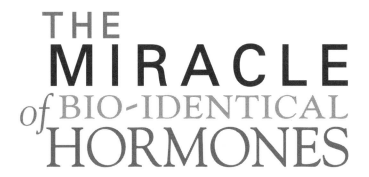

THE
MIRACLE
of BIO-IDENTICAL
HORMONES

HOW I LOST MY: FATIGUE, HOT FLASHES, ADHD,
ADD, FIBROMYALGIA, PMS, OSTEOPOROSIS, WEIGHT,
SEXUAL DYSFUNCTION, ANGER, MIGRAINES...

MICHAEL E. PLATT, M.D.

CLANCY LANE PUBLISHING
california

Clancy Lane Publishing
72-785 Frank Sinatra Drive, Suite B
Rancho Mirage, California 92270

Library of Congress Cataloging-in-Publication Data
Platt, Michael E., M.D.
The miracle of bio-identical hormones: how I lost my: fatigue, hot flashes, ADHD, ADD, fibromyalgia, PMS, osteoporosis, weight, sexual dysfunction, anger, migraines... / Michael E. Platt.
p. cm.
ISBN: 978-0-9776683-2-8
1. Hormone Therapy 2. Health 3. Medicine
I. Title
2007902535

Printed in the United States of America
10 9 8 7 6 5 4 3 2 1
Second Edition

This book is printed on acid-free paper

DESIGNED BY JESSICA STEVENS www.design-savvy.com

NOTE TO THE READER

Please be advised that this book contains my own views and approaches to various medical conditions in men, women, and children.

It is based on years of clinical observation and feedback from my patients, and is tempered by intuition and logic.

This book is not a substitute for any treatment prescribed by your physician.

Any recommendations made in this book should be discussed with your physician, who can order any necessary laboratory evaluations and follow your progress, making adjustments in your treatment as required.

Hormones and how to balance hormones varies from person to person. Although natural bio-identical hormones are safe, their misuse can produce adverse effects or consequences for which the author and publisher cannot be responsible.

This book is not a medical textbook. However, it may provide you with enough information to guide you to wellness with the aid of your physician.

— MICHAEL E. PLATT, M.D.

This book is dedicated to my mother,

Bernice Platt,

whose lifelong battle with hormonal imbalance
ultimately led to her untimely death
at the age of 61 of breast cancer
and belatedly sparked my interest in
natural bio-identical hormones

Doctors give drugs of which they know little
into bodies of which they know less
for diseases of which they know nothing at all.

VOLTAIRE

CONTENTS

FOREWORD

In 1962, when I graduated from Long Island University Brooklyn College of Pharmacy, botany (the study of plants) and pharmacognosy (the medicine of plants) were still being taught. Compounding pharmaceuticals was part of the mainstream curriculum. Then a new course was introduced, which centered on the blending of pharmacy, physiology, and medicine.

With a strong background in a natural pharmaceutical approach to wellness, I was unprepared for the realities of traditional medical approaches to drug therapy.

However, in 1979 I met an amazing physician who renewed my faith in the patient-pharmacist-physician interrelationship. That physician is Michael E. Platt, M.D., a board-certified internist.

At that time in his career he was involved with a number of long-term care facilities where his interest in anti-aging was ignited and his belief in preventive medicine was reinforced. I was servicing the pharmaceutical needs of a number of the same facilities where Dr. Platt was attending. I had immediately taken note that at a time when the national average of drugs for nursing home residents was nine per patient, his patients were on almost no drugs.

When we both moved to Palm Desert, California, within a year of each other, we were able to reestablish the previous three-way patient-pharmacist-physician relationship.

The results once again have been amazing. Dr. Platt's individual approach in treating his patients has rejuvenated my faith in the interplay of the pharmacist and physician in patient care. I was able to witness firsthand the metamorphosis of his patients from sickness to wellness.

As before, he eliminates drugs where possible and continues to focus on preventive medicine. His approach to healing never ceases to amaze me as well as my full-time staff of five pharmacists.

On behalf of my many family members whom he has unselfishly cared for and the many mutual patients we share and help:

Thank you, thank you, thank you.

MORT FARINA, R.Ph.
compounding pharmacist,
Palm Desert, California

ACKNOWLEDGMENTS

Many people have contributed to the making of this book. I will attempt to provide credit to them as due.

My wife, Victoria, has always been my strongest supporter and advocate. More than anyone, she has instilled in me how important it is to share my wellness thoughts with the world. Her insight, feedback, and prodding have kept this book alive.

I thank my best friend, Mort Farina, a compounding pharmacist, whose support I have treasured and who has made it easy for me to achieve wellness in my patients.

I received invaluable assistance from Joyce Sunila, who interviewed the patients and contributed to the format and editing of the book.

My close associate Theresa Quintero spent hours transcribing my scribbling into a coherent form.

Jodene Lloyd, my office manager, helped to facilitate the final birth throes of this book—expeditiously, efficiently, and uncomplainingly.

WJ Carrel, my book shepherd and publicist, has provided ceaseless energy, important insight, and gentle guidance, helping to bring this book to public awareness.

My graphic designer, Jessica Stevens, contributed her admirable talents toward the cover design as well as enhanced the book's readability.

I owe a great deal to Carolyn Bond, whose exceptional expertise as my editor resulted in a book eminently more readable and coherent.

Although I do not know her personally, I must also give Suzanne Somers some credit for this book. The main thrust of my book was finished several years ago—and I did nothing with it until Ms. Somers' book *The Sexy Years* was published. After reading it, I realized that women had to be made aware of an alternative approach to hormone replacement besides the one she proposed. This was my strongest incentive to publish this book.

However, the most important acknowledgment I would like to give is to the thousands of my patients who have provided me with insight and feedback, allowing me to learn how to help them.

WHAT ARE
BIO-IDENTICAL HORMONES?

Bio-identical hormones are hormone supplements whose biochemical structures are identical to those produced by the human body—a fact that offers important therapeutic advantages and minimizes potential risks.

Bio-identical hormones are initially prepared as powders by pharmaceutical companies, such as Upjohn and Pfizer, from a natural base, usually soy or yam. They are FDA-approved. The powders are then sent to compounding pharmacies, where they are formulated according to doctors' prescriptions. Companies like Upjohn have been manufacturing bio-identical hormone products for 70 years.

An exceptionally important advantage of utilizing bio-identical hormones is that dosages can be tailored to the individual's unique hormonal requirements.

Oral bio-identical supplements go directly to the liver, which converts them into a different hormone. Thus the preferred method of delivery for bio-identical hormones is transdermal—in the form of creams, gels, and suppositories—so the hormones are absorbed directly into the bloodstream.

WHY THIS BOOK?

CHAPTER ONE

My name is Michael E. Platt, M.D. I am a board-certified internist with a practice devoted mainly to natural hormone replacement, along with wellness and metabolic weight control. I am writing this book to offer the benefit of my 35 years of clinical experience to people who are unaware of the importance of balanced hormones for health and well-being.

My fundamental approach to illness has always been from the standpoint of dealing with its cause. Since hormones control every system of the body, it is easy to see how foundational they are to people's health. Giving a woman some Motrin for menstrual cramps may relieve the pain, but giving her the correct natural hormone prevents the cramps in the first place. In this book I will be dealing with a wide range of health problems that can be attributed to hormone imbalance—menopause, diabetes, asthma, obesity, migraine headaches, fibromyalgia, arthritis, cancer, fibroids, endometriosis, ADHD (attention deficit hyperactivity disorder), and more.

Hormones are exceptionally powerful substances that have the ability to make you well or make you ill. They affect every cell in the body. It is fairly easy to appreciate the importance of natural rather than synthetic hormones in terms of health maintenance, so it may be a surprise to readers that most doctors have almost no knowledge of natural hormones. Almost everything doctors learn in medical school is based on research done by pharmaceutical companies. Drug companies cannot patent natural products and thereby have no interest in spending hundreds of millions of dollars evaluating natural hormones for which they cannot receive a patent. Most endocrinologists, who specialize in hormones, are familiar with the synthetic hormone compounds produced by drug companies; few of them utilize natural hormones because no drug companies recommend them. Contrary to what many doctors think, bio-identical hormones are obtained in the form of powders from pharmaceutical companies, such as Upjohn and Pfizer, and are FDA approved.

I take a non-traditional approach to medicine because I deal with the cause of disease rather than the symptoms. Some people might say that I practice "alternative" medicine. However, since I utilize natural bio-identical hormones, which match the hormones the body produces, I believe I am practicing "real" medicine. One might argue that those doctors who use synthetic drugs to treat patients are the ones practicing "alternative" medicine. The term "bio-identical" when applied to hormones simply means that the entire hormone is molecularly identical to the hormone produced by the body. And all bio-identical hormones have a natural base, most commonly soy or yam. They can be obtained by prescription from a pharmacy that is specially equipped to formulate and dispense compounded medications—that is, a compounding pharmacy. The number of compounding pharmacies around the country is on the increase.

THE NEW (NOT SO IMPROVED) MEDICINE

The whole idea of preventing disease makes sense to most people—who can argue with it? In the old days, HMOs such as Kaiser and Ross-Loos (the first HMO in the country) were specifically designed to provide preventive health care. In the early 1970s I worked for both organizations at various times. In those days, every lab test and procedure was covered, every medication available was on their formularies, and I was seeing only one patient per hour. Initially, HMOs were run by physicians who understood patient care. Somewhere along the way, insurance companies took over; preventive medicine was eliminated and "managed care" took its place. This perhaps was their way of saying, "What's the least amount of money we can spend and still keep the patient alive?" It's a situation that neither doctors nor patients like, and pretty soon even the insurance companies won't like it as they too become more and more legislated.

With the intervention of the insurance companies, medicine began to change. Increasing specialization eroded the status of family practice. Insurance companies drove up prices while clamping down on the availability of lab tests. I came to feel that medicine was failing to serve the public. In particular, patients' access to appropriate preventive medicine was being sidetracked. Expensive procedures, which yield higher profits than simple remedies, became the standard of practice. Huge capital outlays were made for purchasing the latest medical equipment, which then had to be justified—and sure enough, patients somehow ended up "needing" to utilize the equipment. Doctors became technologists. They lost interest in natural, non-invasive procedures.

Another change was that pharmaceutical companies began funding most of the major medical studies, which are published in medical journals. Thus the pharmaceutical companies began having a lot of say in what doctors read about and also what they are trained to do in medical school. The drug companies' motive for underwriting these studies was not altruistic. It was part of a strategy for market dominance, similar to what happens in any other big business.

However, this book is not intended to be an exposé of American medicine. My purpose is to offer a logical and sensible approach to treating various conditions that differs from traditional practices. Along the way, the book provides a basic understanding of how the body operates, so the reader can understand why something has gone wrong, along with how to fix it.

My observations and advice in this book are based on 35 years of clinical practice. Therefore, you won't find footnotes or a bibliography or references to "double-blind" studies. None of the information here is secret, but much of it is revolutionary. Many doctors today are finding the same faults with conventional medical practice that I have found. A groundswell is starting that, I believe, will, in the next ten years, profoundly alter the way doctors go about treating patients. Most of these changes will be brought about by unhappy yet informed patients who will be asking their physicians to treat their conditions by balancing their hormones utilizing natural bio-identical protocols.

WHAT ABOUT MENOPAUSE?

Perhaps the most controversial, mystifying, and inadequately approached area of medicine today is hormone replacement therapy (HRT). Only relatively recently have women come to question the safety of estrogen and other hormones whose usage has been entrenched in medicine for the past 40 years.

Estrogen can cause aggressive cancers, heart attacks, strokes, and more. In light of recent studies, particularly the Women's Health Initiative of 1997 to 2002, women are being advised to "discuss their individual needs with their health care practitioners." However, all too often the physicians know little more than their patients. If they were well-informed about hormone replacement therapy, especially estrogen replacement therapy (ERT), they might never have prescribed these drugs in the first place. Often the best advice these doctors can give women is: "Don't worry about it," or "The benefits outweigh the risks," or they hand the issue back to the patient: "It's your decision."

Into this wasteland of limited knowledge has walked a new lineup of hormone gurus who propose new alternatives. For the first time women are becoming aware of bio-identical hormones. However, there is a tremendous misconception: that the term "bio-identical" equates with the term "safe." Nothing can be further from the truth. I devote an entire chapter to the correct use of bio-identical hormones for relief of menopausal and perimenopausal problems.

SOMETHING IS WRONG

I am concerned that estrogen is still being prescribed frequently, even though it is associated with six different cancers. It is recommended for patients with osteoporosis, yet there are no studies to show that it benefits women with osteoporosis. It is recommended to help prevent heart disease, yet the last five major studies demonstrate higher incidences of stroke and heart attack while taking estrogen. And don't forget, estrogen is lipogenic: it creates fat and cellulite.

I am concerned that the primary drugs prescribed to treat osteoporosis are also a common reason why people are referred to gastroenterologists; they have toxic side effects on the gastro-intestinal tract. I am concerned that the number one drug being given to prevent recurrence of breast cancer, a drug currently being used by about 700,000 women, has never been adequately demonstrated as effective for breast cancer prevention.

I am concerned that doctors may be blaming the wrong hormone for prostate cancer—a condition that ultimately affects most men if they live long enough. In the course of the book I address these issues and concerns. With the correct approach to hormone replacement, all of them can become non-issues.

LISTENING

One of the most common complaints I hear from patients in my office is that their doctors don't listen to them. When I did my training in medical school, I was taught that 90 percent of a diagnosis is sitting down and talking to the patient. Nowadays, most doctors rush through their day trying to squeeze in as many patients as possible. They don't have time to truly listen. The average time a doctor spends with a patient is four minutes. And even when a doctor does take the time to listen to a patient, he or she still tends to treat the symptoms and not the cause of the problem. So the patient is still not well.

My patients are amazed when, on their first visit, I sit down and talk to them for an hour, delving into not just their own health backgrounds but the health backgrounds of all their family members. I do this for a very good reason: the more I know about my patients' bodies, their genetic history, the medications they have taken in the past, how they have responded to various interventions, and so on, the better I am able to help them. By listening deeply I can detect hormone imbalance in the particulars of people's lives, I can see clues to metabolic problems in certain kinds of behavior. My talks with patients are invaluable. Often, the lab tests that are done afterward merely confirm what I have already inferred from our talk.

A side benefit of the long initial conversation is that my patients develop trust. They feel attended to. Bodies are complex, intricate mechanisms. The only way to understand them is in depth. My patients sense the rightness in my probing deeply into their health backgrounds. Conversely, they sense something is wrong when a doctor dismisses them after a four-minute discussion and dispenses a one-size-fits-all treatment. They feel discounted.

The medical community has, in my opinion, become complacent. By and large, we physicians are not showing a deep personal commitment to the people who create our livelihoods. We accept all too easily that increasing numbers of our patients are over-weight, that women are having miscarriages and developing breast cancer and other cancers, and that coronary artery disease and other cardiovascular ailments are running rampant. We accept the fact that many of our patients are taking multiple medications with a range of unpleasant side effects. Prescription drugs are known to be the second leading cause of death; I suspect they may actually be the primary.

Our patients are suffering, and in many cases their suffering is preventable. But before we can treat them at the causal level and ease their suffering, we must learn to listen.

HOW THIS BOOK IS ORGANIZED

Throughout this book you will be meeting some of my patients, hearing how they felt when they first came to my office and how they felt after being restored to health. As you read their case histories you'll see how I managed to heal ailments that had been dogging them for years just by balancing their hormones. Conventional doctors had treated these ailments with prescription drugs, many of which had side effects that brought on more symptoms and more disease. I was able to halt this negative progression by bringing the body's own natural endocrine system back into balance.

After my patients tell their stories, I comment on how I conducted their treatment and why they got the results they did. There is a certain amount of overlap across chapters. Most people have multiple hormonal imbalances, so many of my patients share similar clusters of symptoms.

> *I see many protocols in medicine today that aren't in the patients' best interest, and the public's only defense against these practices is awareness.*

Besides the case histories, there are other chapters that offer simple, non-technical explanations of a variety of topics. For instance, while discussing weight management, I talk about medications that cause weight gain and the thyroid supplements that do and don't work to regulate metabolism, that is, I present information that may help readers find the key to their own weight management. In another chapter I put the topic of cholesterol into perspective in a similar way. I see many protocols in medicine today that aren't in the patients' best interest, and the public's only defense against these practices is awareness.

There is, of course, an important chapter on bio-identical hormone treatment of menopause in women. Another chapter discusses bio-identical hormones and andropause in men. Armed with this information, patients should be able to question their doctors and insist on proper care. One of my purposes in writing this book is to help those pro-active, intelligent readers—and I know there are many of you out there, far more than when I first started practicing—who take pride in being conscientious, informed medical consumers.

Patients have often told me that what I say is different from anything they've heard prior to coming to me. They have often encouraged: "Doc, you should write a book."

Well, this is that book. I cannot prove any of the opinions I'm putting forth here in a way that would satisfy the demands of objective science, such as double-blind studies—but I know they are sound enough to consistently create results for my patients. Perhaps in time they'll be shown to have the scientific backing I can't claim for them today. Drs. Semmelweiss and Lister were ridiculed in their day for suggesting that doctors wash their hands and wear gloves prior to operating on patients. They were telling doctors that they were infecting their patients, but very few believed this. Doctors, like most people, resist change.

AMAZING HORMONES

Many people are amazed to find that balancing hormones has such wide-ranging effects on patients' health. But why not? Hormones regulate every aspect of our physical being. For the various hormones our bodies produce there are thousands of receptor sites distributed all over the body. Each kind of receptor site has the power to alter the body's behavior in profound ways.

I believe the benefits of natural bio-identical hormone therapy should be available to everyone, and this book is designed to teach the reading public about those benefits. I am not writing this book for doctors, although I would welcome their readership. I am speaking to the public directly because

I've observed again and again how people committed to their own health can change the system. In the past 35 years I've seen dozens of "unconventional" medical solutions brought into the mainstream by patients who insisted that doctors (and insurance companies) should give them what they want. Acupuncture, herbal remedies, meditation, and other "fringe" ideas have bubbled up into popular consciousness and earned credibility. I would like to see natural hormones come into the mainstream in the same way. By writing this book, I hope to join the chorus of voices focusing attention on natural bio-identical hormone therapy.

PERMANENT WEIGHT LOSS

I have placed the weight loss chapter toward the end of this book for a very good reason. I don't think the world needs another diet book. I don't want this book to be confused in any way with a diet book. Delaying my weight management theory until late in the book is a way of asking that the reader develop an understanding of hormones before embarking on my weight loss approach.

The reader who skips the information in the early chapters of this book, intent only on finding out how to lose weight, may be disappointed. There is nothing in chapter 20 that can help the reader lose weight until he or she understands the role of hormones in regulating metabolic health.

As you will see when you get to that chapter, I have a very different approach to permanent weight loss. Simply cutting out "carbs" is not the answer. I have observed that for many patients, no matter what they do to lose weight, sooner or later it comes back on again. Why? Because no one has helped them deal with the underlying reasons for weight gain in the first place.

Ninety-nine percent of the time there is a hormonal problem. Keep in mind that hormones control every system of the body—including metabolism, which factors into weight. The majority of people with weight problems produce too much insulin. In these cases, reducing carbohydrates is mandatory. This is not a new concept—as of this writing, it is 157 years old. It is the basic approach utilized by the Atkins Diet, Sugar Busters, the South Beach Diet, the Carbohydrate Addicts Diet, Protein Power, and others. What makes my approach different is that I address the underlying reason why the body is producing excess insulin. Without this, the fat comes right back after the person discontinues the low-carb meal plan. This book's approach to weight, then, is actually a step beyond the Atkins or the South Beach diet.

FINDING MY AUDIENCE

I find it impossible to fit my ideas into pat formulas. This book is not a diet book or a self-help book, although it does contain elements that should be useful to people seeking both kinds of books. What you will find here is a strong point of view about the role of natural hormones in restoring and maintaining wellness, along with some thoughts about the state of the health care industry at this time.

My hope is that serendipity will bring this book to the people who need it most. I offer some guidelines on how to use hormones with the help of your doctor. A prescription can be obtained and filled at a compounding pharmacy. I don't publish food lists, menus, tables (such as the glycemic index), and so on. These aids to the daily process of planning healthy meals can be found in other books. My goal here is to set forth basic principles.

"IT CAN'T BE THAT EASY"

Often after I've talked to a patient about their lifelong medical problem and outlined a course of treatment, the patient responds—sometimes teary-eyed—"Doc, it can't be that easy." They've gone from doctor to doctor; they've read book after book. Many find me in the second half of their life—their quest has gone on that long.

The tragedy is that it *is* that easy. Today's medical model has turned health care into a complex, expensive enterprise. Specialists treat symptoms with great technical wizardry and pharmacological sophistication—while ignoring causes. Behind all the sound and fury lies a simple, overlooked truth: bodies in hormonal balance can reach a level of optimum health in a natural manner.

PLEASE NOTE

In this book, whenever I use the term "natural" for hormones, I am referring only to bio-identical hormones. Any hormone described as "natural" may not always be bio-identical; for example, Premarin is technically natural, since it is made from a natural substance (pregnant mares' urine), but it is not bio-identical. "Bio-identical" means the hormone supplement has the same biochemical structure as the hormone made by the human body.

ESTROGEN DOMINANCE
AND BRENDA J.

CHAPTER TWO

Brenda J., 57, visited my office primarily to discuss a weight problem. As we talked, it became clear that her "bloat," as she called it, was actually a minor factor in a constellation of symptoms whose roots were hormonal. Far more serious than her weight were complaints that had begun surfacing when she was in her late 20s and thereafter accelerated rapidly: an inability to focus, constant headaches, chronic fatigue, aching bones and joints, and disorientation.

I am going to let Brenda tell her story, after which I'll answer the questions you might ask if we were at a workshop together and you wanted to understand how I treated Brenda. I'll explain how unbalanced hormones hurt her and how balancing her hormones healed her. I believe her situation is not uncommon. Readers with similar afflictions may see something of themselves in the way Brenda experienced a 30-year bout with estrogen dominance.

I've had a lot of female problems since I was very, very young. My first child was born when I was 17 years old. Paul was born a severe quadriplegic with cerebral palsy. When I was 18, my second child was born and died after three months. At 22, my daughter, Sandra, was born. She was normal but very, very tiny: three pounds. All of my children were born prematurely.

When I was 23 I had to have a complete hysterectomy. I had fibroid tumors, and one night I went into a very severe hemorrhage and was taken to the emergency room where doctors performed the hysterectomy.

Estrogen replacement was recommended by my gynecologist after the hysterectomy. I was told I would need to take estrogen for the rest of my life, since my body no longer produced it.

As soon as I began taking Premarin I felt that something was wrong. I just didn't feel right. I told my gynecologist about this feeling and I suggested it might be the estrogen. But he told me that wasn't the problem and that I had to be on estrogen. That was when I began gaining weight.

For the first five years after my hysterectomy my only symptom was this gradual weight gain. But then other symptoms began appearing. I began feeling fuzzy in the head. My vision started to blur, I wasn't sleeping well and my joints started hurting.

When my first gynecologist retired, another doctor took over his practice. I tried talking to this doctor too, telling him how I felt. But he had the same response to my complaints as the first doctor. In fact, he thought my symptoms indicated that I might not be getting enough estrogen and he increased my dosage. This doctor put me on Synthroid, a thyroid drug, and kept increasing the amount of Premarin I was taking, so that by the time I was in my 40s I'd been taking 2.5 mg, the maximum dosage of Premarin, for 10 or 12 years. The gynecologist would explain away my depression by saying, "Of course you're depressed. You have a handicapped child. You had a child that died. Your depression is normal."

I got divorced in my 30s, and about a year after the divorce my physical problems started in earnest: the aches and pains, the fuzzy thinking, the deep fatigue, the headaches, and of course the bloated body, which got worse every year. I honestly don't know how I managed back in those days after the divorce. I was so exhausted all the time I didn't know which end was up.

A typical day would start with my getting up and my body hurting so badly that I would get into the shower and stand under the hot water until I could bend my arms and legs and move a little. Then I would get dressed and I was already exhausted. But somehow I'd do my work; you just do what you have to do.

During this whole time I tried getting second, third, and fourth opinions about the Premarin from various gynecologists. When I moved to Lake Arrowhead, California, I tried a gynecologist there. This doctor told me to keep taking the Premarin and that the only problem I had with weight was that I had to stop eating so much. I told him, "I don't eat. I starve myself to death and I exercise until I fall on my face and almost pass out." He said, "Well, I never saw a fat woman in a concentration camp." I got so mad I got up and walked out of his office. Shortly after that I read about this program at Duke University where you could get a total medical workup. I flew to Raleigh, North Carolina, and entered the program. I filled out endless forms and had blood tests and a hormone panel and all kinds of testing done. I lived there for six weeks and spent almost $20,000.

At the end of the whole thing they told me there was nothing wrong with me and that I should go home and visit a psychiatrist. It was the same old song: you've had a hard life, you're stressed out, keep taking your Premarin and see a counselor.

The doctors at Duke University increased my dosage of Synthroid and put me on a high-carbohydrate diet. I was eating bagels and fruit in the morning, pasta for lunch and dinner, and now I started really bloating out. My metabolism was slowing down even more. I have photographs of myself from this period, and it takes my breath away to look at them. I was so huge! I was a size 14.

I developed a new symptom. I started having disoriented moments when I'd be on the freeway and I couldn't remember where I was going or why I was there.

The turnaround came when I talked to a woman who was having some of the same problems I was having—achy joints, weight gain, puffiness, fatigue. We'd commiserate with each other, blaming it on our age. "Getting old isn't what it's cracked up to be," we'd tell each other. I didn't see her for about four or five months, and then one day I was out walking my dog and ran into her. I hardly recognized her. "My God, what are you doing?" I asked. She told me about Dr. Platt, and I went to see him the following week.

The first thing I noticed about Dr. Platt was that he really listened to me. Most doctors don't hear you, but Dr. Platt makes you feel like you're talking to your best friend. He did my hormone panel and told me he was taking me off Premarin. My first reaction was shock. All of my life doctors had been telling me that I needed estrogen replacement. I thought, "Maybe this isn't going to work." A few times I'd tried to wean myself from Premarin, and the hot flashes and headaches were unbearable.

And the way he was telling me to eat! Meats and vegetables, bacon and eggs for breakfast—it went against everything the culture was telling us about cholesterol and everything else. But at the end of our first meeting he said something that made me trust him. He said, "None of this is your fault. You've just never received proper treatment."

So I started taking progesterone, two different thyroid hormones, and eating what he told me to eat. I was eating meat, eating eggs, eating three meals a day. I never ate so much in my life. And the results happened so fast I couldn't believe it. I could just see the weight dropping daily. And my energy shot up. I don't ever remember feeling the way I started to feel. I felt wonderful and happy and energetic.

I can't even describe it, it all happened so fast. I was thinking clearly, my vision cleared up, my headaches stopped, I started sleeping at night. In about a month I had to buy a new wardrobe. I immediately got rid of everything in size 14. I went down to a size 4 in two months.

The aches and pains started going away gradually. At six months I realized that my arms didn't hurt. I could get up in the morning and move my arms.

By this time I felt so great that my new husband couldn't keep up with me. I had more energy than he could handle. So he went to see Dr. Platt, and he got amazing results, too. He's 11 years older than me and has always been very healthy, but now he feels like 40 again.

When I see friends, they're shocked at how well I look. They think I've lost 90 pounds (I've actually only lost 47 pounds). My vitality is unlike anything they've seen in me before.

You know, when it comes right down to it, it isn't even the difference in how you look ... it is how you feel. I wouldn't give up how I feel for anything.

MIRACLE OR SIMPLE CHEMISTRY?

The transformation Brenda J. testifies to may sound incredible, but the truth is that it's not an unusual occurrence in my practice. I attribute every bit of it to the power of hormones. They regulate activity in every cell in the body, including the brain cells. As miraculous as Brenda's healing sounds, it was no miracle—it was a matter of chemistry, pure and simple.

When Brenda first came to see me, she showed all the classic signs of estrogen dominance. She'd been laboring under the burden of excess estrogen her entire life, even before she was prescribed estrogen in the form of Premarin in her 20s. The reason for her over-production of estrogen was a lack of progesterone. This deficiency of progesterone was the major cause of her problem pregnancies, and certainly the cause of her fibroids, which ultimately resulted in the need for a hysterectomy.

Just putting her on natural bio-identical progesterone made her feel better right away. Progesterone is a natural anti-depressant; it's the feel-good hormone for women. With the proper amount of progesterone in her body, Brenda's mood brightened. Progesterone is the hormone that balances out estrogen and takes away its worst side effects.

Progesterone is also thermogenic. It helps fat to burn by helping the thyroid gland to function better, as well as by raising body temperature. And it helps prevent the over-production of insulin, the main hormone that creates fat and keeps it stored. So Brenda's metabolism improved and she began to see her weight melting away.

She was more comfortable inside her own body. That alone had to make her feel much, much better. Her fatigue started lifting, too. She had energy she hadn't had before.

Part of her weight loss was related to a reduction in the fluid retention caused by too much estrogen, too much insulin, and the wrong thyroid medication.

THE UNFRIENDLY EFFECTS OF ESTROGEN

The improvement I saw in Brenda just a month or two after starting her on progesterone is something I see again and again in my practice. People have to understand that in many cases estrogen is toxic to the body. You can think of progesterone as an anti-estrogen hormone. Progesterone is there to protect the body from the negative effects of estrogen.

Which negative effects? Estrogen is very damaging to blood vessels. This is why it causes migraine headaches. Doctors are very much aware of estrogen's effect on blood vessels. It's why they warn women on birth control pills to be on the lookout for signs of phlebitis, which is an inflammation of the veins. Birth control pills contain two synthetic hormones—an estrogen and a progestin. (Progestin is a synthetic form of progesterone. It is a chemical that is unrelated to natural progesterone and has the same side effects as estrogen.)

Estrogen causes six different cancers in women. It's been known for over 50 years that estrogen causes breast cancer. To my knowledge, estrogen and the drug Tamoxifen are the only known causes of cancer of the uterus. Estrogen is also a cause of ovarian cancer, cervical cancer, vaginal cancer, and cancer of the colon.

For years an effort was made to place estrogen on the list of cancer-causing chemicals. Once a drug is on this list, special warnings are supposed to be given. Estrogen was finally put on this list in 2003; however, you wouldn't know it because it is never mentioned.

Morning sickness is only caused by too much estrogen. But doctors don't realize that. They don't know that you can prevent morning sickness and also prevent miscarriages by prescribing bio-identical progesterone. Natural hormones can help women with common problems like these, but doctors are generally unaware of it.

Estrogen has always been promoted for the treatment of osteoporosis, and it appears that in some studies it may prevent osteoporosis temporarily. Yet there have been no studies to show that estrogen reverses osteoporosis. In fact, it is primarily a lack of progesterone that causes osteoporosis. Studies are now finding that women on birth control pills, which suppress progesterone production, have an earlier onset of osteoporosis.

In women, progesterone is one of the hormones of choice in the treatment of osteoporosis. It stimulates osteoblasts in the bone to make new bone. Estrogen does not do this.

STANDING UP TO ESTROGEN DOMINANCE

I am not the first doctor to point out the over-use of estrogen in medicine today. The term "estrogen dominance" was coined by Dr. John R. Lee in his 1996 book, *What Your Doctor May Not Tell You about Menopause.* He was the first physician to go public decrying the use of estrogen to "cure" women's menopause.

Unfortunately, the concept of estrogen dominance is not widely accepted in the medical community—a result of the fact that many doctors have very little understanding of hormones at all. This is a point I'll come back to again and again. It's one of the primary themes of this book: the conventional medical community is largely unaware of how important hormones are in regulating every aspect of our physical well being; or rather, they understand its importance intellectually but do not apply this in their practices.

Most doctors were never taught in medical school that a person can have too much estrogen. To the medical community there's no such thing as a disease caused by too much estrogen. They know that there are conditions called fibroids and endometriosis, they know that women get fibrocystic disease in their breasts and so on, but they don't seem concerned about estrogen's role in causing these conditions. Women with these problems should never be given estrogen because they are at risk for even more serious complications from estrogen dominance.

It is very difficult for people, doctors included, to separate the hype associated with estrogen from the reality. Most of the research on estrogen has been bought and paid for by drug companies, who have almost 100 percent control over what gets published and, more importantly, what doesn't.

It's long been proposed by drug companies, and therefore by the doctors who tend to believe what these companies have to say, that estrogen is good for the heart. Yet five recent major studies have indicated that women starting on estrogen have higher incidences of heart attacks and strokes. For this reason, estrogen is now contra-indicated for women with coronary artery disease and women who have had strokes. Another negative side effect of estrogen is that it elevates levels of homocysteine, the substance that makes blood vessels sticky, leading to clot and plaque formation. The American Heart Association is now telling doctors to be much more selective in giving women estrogen.

This is a good place to make a comment about the term "estrogen" as it is used throughout the book. There are three basic types of estrogen: estradiol, estrone, and estriol, listed here from the strongest to the weakest. Estradiol is the one associated with most of the unpleasant side effects women experience, as well as the hormonal cancers that occur in both men and women. (However, using it transdermally appears to provide a level of safety in this regard.) Accordingly, when I mention the negative aspects of estrogen, I am usually referring to estradiol.

Estriol, the weakest and thereby the safest estrogen, does not cause cancerous changes in the cells. In fact, it is so safe that it has been used to treat breast cancer, since it occupies estrogen receptor sites and blocks stronger forms of estrogen. It is also the best type of estrogen for vaginal dryness.

Transdermal estrogens, even estradiol when applied transdermally, are basically safer than estrogens taken orally. However, they should never be used without concomitant progesterone cream to counteract the estrogen and avoid potential side effects. And keep in mind that all estrogens are lipogenic—they all create fat.

THE HEALING POWERS OF PROGESTERONE

When you realize that there are over 300 receptor sites for progesterone throughout the body, you can begin to appreciate the powerful effects patients can experience when they are given this hormone.

In general, progesterone is wonderful for brain tissue. In fact, progesterone levels are higher in brain tissue than anywhere else in the body. So progesterone influences memory function, and some studies indicate that it's very good for preventing and possibly even treating Alzheimer's disease.

Progesterone is also wonderful for nerve tissue. I've used it with diabetics who have a burning neuropathy in their feet. Sometimes the neuropathy is gone within three days. Progesterone also stimulates the Schwann cells that line the axis of a nerve and produce myelin. Multiple sclerosis (MS) is a condition associated with the demyelinization of nerve cells. Most of the patients with MS who I have treated have been estrogen dominant. Could this condition possibly be related to low progesterone levels?

Progesterone also has a healing effect on blood vessels. It undoes all the damage that estrogen causes. That's why it works so well for preventing and treating menstrual migraines, and why it's effective in preventing coronary artery spasm.

One of the best treatments for osteoporosis happens to be progesterone. It's much better than estrogen in this regard. And because progesterone reduces the level of insulin—the number one hormone that causes the accumulation of fat in most people—it can be used to help control weight.

Being a feel-good hormone, especially for women, progesterone is also a natural anti-depressant. As the antidote to estrogen, it helps prevent breast cancer, cancer of the ovaries, and probably cancer of the colon. In my view, it can also prevent cancer of the prostate, which I believe is another cancer caused by estrogen.

Brenda would have had a completely different life if the benefits of progesterone had been understood by the medical community. Instead, she was estrogen dominant, which led to her hysterectomy and brought on a surgically induced menopause. At that point, Brenda became a victim of the Premarin trend, also known as estrogen replacement therapy (ERT), which began in earnest in the 1970s. Before the 1970s, there was nothing in the gynecological canon that dictated giving women estrogen at menopause. I discuss the story of Premarin and ERT in chapter 10, the chapter on menopause and perimenopause.

FIBROMYALGIA

The pain that Brenda began to experience in her 30s was due to fibromyalgia. In my practice I come across many patients in whom physical pain—arthritis, fibromyalgia, and so forth—is intermixed with symptoms of hormone imbalance. Just getting their hormones in balance often leads to relief. Those hormones most often involved include progesterone, insulin, adrenaline, cortisol, and thyroid.

For the most part, these people are angry. Their hormone imbalances are allowed to go on year after year. They take part in expensive, time-consuming efforts to treat their symptoms, and the symptoms stubbornly persist. It's understandable that they'd develop anger about their lot in life. I've found fibromyalgia to be present in many of the people who seek out my services, and, as with Brenda, it usually has not been properly diagnosed.

Anger can cause muscles to tense. When you tense a muscle, it produces lactic acid which causes pain, and the persistent tensing of the muscles utilizes a lot of energy, which causes fatigue.

Although Brenda doesn't mention it in her story, she told me during her intake interview that she was also operated on for TMJ, or pain in the temporomandibular joint. TMJ is caused by tensing of the jaw muscles, which occurs usually at night and is always associated with anger. Brenda had a lot of good reasons to be angry. She was being misled by the medical community, and she had—let's face it—a hard life raising her children on her own. I find her situation almost tragic. She was crying out for help, exhibiting classic symptoms that should have been impossible to miss, yet no one would listen to her.

In chapter 7 I discuss the way I treat patients with fibromyalgia, which is to deal with the underlying cause of their anger and to get their hormones back in balance.

> *If you can balance a patient's hormones,*
> *you can often treat their problems at the source*
> *without resorting to surgery and drugs.*

I cannot emphasize enough the importance of utilizing hormones correctly. Some women are more sensitive to foreign substances than others. Brenda was a woman who sensed something wrong the moment Premarin was introduced into her system. She communicated this to her doctor, but he refused to give credence to her intuition. Ironically, when she tried to wean herself off Premarin, she suffered hot flashes and headaches. This is because foreign substances, once they are established on the cellular level, are difficult to flush out. For many women, coming off Premarin is like coming off heroin. A woman may go through severe withdrawal headaches, nausea, hot flashes, night sweats, and so on in the process.

The hot flashes and night sweats may be caused by luteinizing hormone (LH), a hormone secreted by the pituitary gland. The pituitary sends this hormone to stimulate the ovaries to produce more estrogen, progesterone, or other hormones. Anything that elevates luteinizing hormone—a lack of estrogen, progesterone, and perhaps even testosterone—will produce the vasomotor effects that women get, that is, hot flashes and night sweats. Thus taking someone off estrogen can precipitate hot flashes. Or sometimes the pituitary is reacting to the fact that progesterone is low. So just giving progesterone can take away hot flashes.

In another chapter I address how to wean someone off of Premarin. As you can see, balancing a person's hormones is a delicate juggling act.

WHY DUKE UNIVERSITY MEDICAL CENTER FAILED BRENDA J.

The medical center at Duke University is one of the most respected in the world. Brenda went there and told them she just didn't feel good, so they put her through $20,000 worth of testing and at the end of six weeks said, basically, "There's nothing wrong with you. You have to speak to a psychiatrist."

How could this happen? How could a major medical research center fail to diagnose someone properly after $20,000 worth of tests?

One of the reasons is something I witness over and over again among conventional doctors: they don't treat patients, they treat lab tests. Few doctors sit down and talk to patients any more. If the doctors at Duke had taken the time with Brenda, it would have been hard for them to miss the constellation of symptoms she was exhibiting.

Moreover, when most doctors do blood tests, they don't always test for hormones. If they do, they don't always test for the correct hormones. I have worked with enough cases of hormone imbalance that even before seeing the results of Brenda's blood tests, I knew that she was suffering from estrogen dominance and hypothyroidism, her symptoms were so classic.

It's not surprising to me that a medical center like Duke could miss Brenda's symptomatology. The doctors at Duke University are no doubt good doctors. However, most of them are academically inclined and simply won't consider non-traditional approaches that have not been verified by double-blind studies. Universities, and the hospitals and clinics associated with them, tend toward medical conservatism. They're also heavily influenced by pharmaceutical companies, which fund all the big medical research studies, creating an aura of legitimacy around their products. In these settings, doctors' view of the wellness movement and natural products is skewed. They tend to dismiss both.

AN UNDER-ACTIVE THYROID

Excess estrogen and low progesterone weren't Brenda's only hormone problems. She also had an under-active thyroid. Once her body received the correct type and dose of thyroid supplement, her metabolism increased and she was able to burn fat. She had more energy. As her fat reserves shrank, she felt lighter and more optimistic.

The doctors at Duke University diagnosed Brenda as having an under-active thyroid, but they used an inappropriate thyroid approach. Doctors, for the most part, fail to realize there are two different thyroid hormones and both have to be assessed. In spite of $20,000 worth of testing, the physicians at Duke did not see that Brenda was not making enough triiodothyronine (T3)—the thyroid hormone responsible for 90 percent of the thyroid's activity. They gave her Synthroid, which is thyroxine (T4), basically a storage hormone. T4 must be converted to T3 to be effective, but Brenda's body was unable to convert T4 into T3, so Synthroid did not help her. I discuss thyroid function and treatment in more detail in chapter 3.

The influence of the pharmaceutical companies is also a factor to some extent here. Synthroid is so well-publicized that it's all that most doctors know when it comes to supplementing the thyroid gland.

Six weeks after her first visit to my office, Brenda came in and we sat down and talked. "Doc," she said, "I've never felt better in my entire life." That shows you the power of hormones.

AN OUNCE OF PREVENTION

To my mind, Brenda's life and her battle with estrogen teach one very important lesson: it's easier to prevent disease than it is to cure it. That's why it's essential that doctors educate themselves about hormones. They're foundational. If you can balance a patient's hormones, you can often treat their problems at the source without resorting to surgery and drugs. Brenda is a perfect example of the miraculous power of bio-identical hormone therapy.

THYROID HORMONES—
TWO TYPES

CHAPTER THREE

The thyroid gland controls metabolism in every cell of the body. A thyroid deficiency can cause a multitude of symptoms, the classic ones being weight gain, dry skin, poor nails, low body temperature, sluggishness, and memory problems. In women, other common symptoms are blood clots during their periods and hair loss. Thyroid hormone controls the rate at which calories are burned to produce energy. Dr. Atkins, originator of the Atkins Diet, has stated that the number one reason for "metabolic resistance"—the term he uses to describe the inability to burn fat—is a thyroid deficiency.

THE WRONG THYROID HORMONE

Although most people don't realize it, there are actually two thyroid hormones, triiodothyronine (T3) and thyroxine (T4). The thyroid gland produces and releases T4, which goes to the liver, where it is converted into T3. T4 does not perform most of the tasks of the thyroid hormone—it is essentially a storage hormone. T3, the active form of thyroid, is responsible for most, but not all, of its functions. Obviously, any problem resulting in a lack of T3 will create low thyroid symptoms.

Unfortunately, in the medical community today, when testing and treating thyroid disorders most doctors test only for T4 and regard it as the barometer of a person's metabolic health. They don't realize that some people can have a perfectly normal T4 level and still be hypothyroid (lacking in sufficient thyroid hormone) because of an inability to convert T4 to T3. Unless their bodies can convert T4 into T3, they will lack the essential ingredient for a properly acting metabolism.

The most commonly prescribed medications for low thyroid conditions are Synthroid, Levoxyl, and levothyroxine. These are T4 preparations—which means that most people who exhibit low thyroid symptoms are being given something that may or may not address their problem. In my practice I constantly come across patients who have been taking Synthroid for years without getting any relief from their hypothyroid symptoms. Their doctors continue to prescribe the T4 preparation despite the lack of results because their blood tests show normal T4 levels. As I've said before, too many doctors treat blood tests instead of patients.

T3 preparations are available, but for the most part they are ignored by the medical community.

Possibly aggravating the problem are any of a number of medications that interfere with thyroid metabolism and prevent or slow the conversion of T4 into T3. These include cholesterol-lowering statin-type drugs such as Lipitor and Zocor. These lower coenzyme Q-10, a factor necessary for thyroid conversion. I talk about these again in chapter 19, which discusses the medications that prevent weight loss.

Ironically, one of the most common reasons for an elevated cholesterol level is an under-active thyroid. This means that people who take statin-type drugs for cholesterol are taking a thyroid-blocking drug to treat a condition that may be caused by an under-active thyroid in the first place. When I see people with high cholesterol, my first thought is that they might be low in thyroid. In fact, in the old days, cholesterol used to be called "the poor man's thyroid test."

Beta-blockers such as atenolol, Ziac, and Lopressor also block the conversion of T4 into T3. These drugs are often prescribed by cardiologists for their heart patients to reduce the workload of the heart. However, they almost guarantee weight gain, which is, ironically, one of the most significant risk factors for coronary artery disease.

THYROID STIMULATING HORMONE

I apologize if the discussion is getting a little long and technical, but one cannot underestimate the importance of knowing about thyroid metabolism. My sense is that millions of people are being improperly treated, or not treated at all, for an under-active thyroid condition. The reasons are twofold: the failure of many doctors to listen to what their patients are saying, and the failure of many doctors to interpret laboratory tests logically.

Most physicians regard the test for TSH, or thyroid stimulating hormone, the most sensitive of all thyroid tests—in fact, it's often the only thyroid test that's ordered. If the pituitary gland detects suboptimal thyroid levels, it sends out TSH to stimulate the thyroid to make more hormones. "Normal" levels of TSH are considered to fall between 0.3 to 5.5. If your TSH level is within this range, your test is considered normal and no thyroid will be prescribed. However, the fact is that any TSH level greater than 1.0 can mean your pituitary is saying "you need thyroid." The normal range was arbitrarily established by determining the TSH levels of 100 medical students, with no concern as to how their thyroids were functioning.

Doctors usually wait to see a TSH level higher than 5.5 before they prescribe treatment. But patients with that high a level are severely hypothyroid. My goal when I treat patients is to get the TSH level close to 0.3, at which point I know they are getting close to 100 percent of the thyroid they require. However, I use two different thyroid hormones to achieve this—both T3 and T4. A low TSH in a patient who is taking only Synthroid or Levoxyl may indicate that they are taking too much of the medication, especially if the patient also shows a higher than normal heart rate.

WHAT YOU CAN DO

A proper thyroid evaluation should include taking the patient's history, looking at the patient, and ordering the proper tests. Signs and symptoms of low thyroid, as I mentioned before, include: dry skin (without using moisturizers), brittle or soft nails, cold feet, blood clots with periods, low body temperature, fatigue, poor memory, dry and brittle hair, elevated cholesterol, and weight gain. Sensible thyroid testing would include:

- Free T4
- Free T3
- TSH

Note: Free T4 and free T3 does not mean there is no fee involved. Rather, "free" refers to thyroid that is unbound and biologically active and so is not affected by levels of thyroid binding globulin.

T3 PREPARATIONS

To my way of thinking, proper thyroid dosing is likely to include both thyroid hormones. There are various T3 preparations, such as Armour, Thyrolar, and Cytomel. The first two are combinations of T3 and T4. However, the T3 is short-acting (three hours), and neither preparation has enough T4. Cytomel is a synthetic T3 and is also short-acting.

My preference is giving a sustained-release form of bio-identical T3 (obtainable only through a compounding pharmacy) to be taken once or twice a day. If the free T3 level is below 280 pg/dl, I prescribe 7.5 mcg of T3-S/R. In addition I prescribe the proper dose of L-thyroxin (Levoxyl or Synthroid), usually 0.125 mg, corresponding to a free T4 level of 1.1 ng/dl.

Note that people with ADHD always have low thyroid levels. They are also low in progesterone, which is required for proper thyroid functioning. If a patient has undiagnosed ADHD (a common occurrence) and the doctor is only treating lab tests and not symptoms (also a common occurrence), the patient may experience uncomfortable side effects, such as palpitations, headache, or a rise in blood pressure, after starting on thyroid. Both adrenaline, which is part of the ADHD causation, and thyroid are stimulants, so ADHD must be treated, by lowering the adrenaline levels, prior to starting thyroid. The decrease in energy level that ADHD patients experience as their adrenaline levels are lowered is balanced again with thyroid, which brings their energy levels back up.

My approach to ADHD is presented in chapter 15.

HORMONAL FATIGUE AND RHONDA Y.

CHAPTER FOUR

Fatigue is a common symptom in bodies that are out of balance. For Rhonda Y., 38, hormonally induced fatigue had eroded the joy of raising her family. Fortunately, I was able to help her regain hormonal balance, restoring her zest for living and ability to have a full life with her loved ones. But how many chronically fatigued homemakers stumble through the daily grind of the caregiver's life, branded as hypochondriacs and failing to receive help?

I've chosen to include Rhonda in this book because I find something frightening in the way the medical system failed her and fails people like her every day. Here is her story:

My medical problems began early, with pains in my pelvic area that would get so bad I would be doubled over. My first pregnancy was an ectopic pregnancy. That's a pregnancy in which the fetus develops in the fallopian tubes, and I had to have surgery for that. Later I had endometriosis and went through several operations for that. My two sons were conceived through the expensive and painful method of in vitro fertilization.

At age 31 my whole system started taking a dive. That was when the weight gain started. My weight had always been normal, but suddenly I started putting on pounds. Along with the weight came a host of new symptoms.

One was asthma. Another was acid reflux, which was very painful, and then came a third painful condition, irritable bowel syndrome. I developed high blood pressure and also had a kidney infection. These were all debilitating conditions, but the worst of it was a new level of fatigue that hit me, that made raising my children a kind of daily torment.

The fatigue went on all day, but it would hit me hard at about 7 or 8 o'clock at night, at which time I just couldn't do anything. I pretty much set my bedtime at 8 P.M. The fatigue made domestic chores impossible to complete. I needed to rest a lot during the day. The messes around the house began to seem like mountains I had to climb. The kids' demands were constant, and I lost my cheerfulness early in the day. I yelled a lot and felt constantly irritable.

Often I couldn't face putting a big meal on the table in the evening and cleaning up afterwards, so I'd take the kids out for fast food. (My husband didn't come home until 8 or 9 o'clock at night.) I was craving caffeine and sugar to give myself a lift, and I could get those at a fast food place. I felt guilty about not giving my kids whole foods, but by the time evening came around I often felt too tired to care. Luckily, I'm blessed with wonderful kids who were aware of my problem and learned how to take care of themselves.

I was just getting by as a mother, doing the bare minimum. The area where there was the most fallout was recreation and social activities. Once I'd taken care of the necessities, I just didn't have the energy for anything more. My husband would take the kids places on Sundays, but I never went with them; I was so relieved just to be able to rest and not have anyone asking me for anything. The kids got used to playing with their dad and not expecting mom to be there.

As far as socializing with other families went, I didn't have what it took to prepare meals and entertain. We were isolated. My husband compensated by socializing with his family, who live close by. I enjoy my husband's family but I rarely went with him and the kids. I just wanted to rest.

I went to a lot of doctors about the fatigue. They all said there was nothing they could do about it. Most of them were condescending and treated me like a child or some kind of mental case.

My husband was constantly concerned about my health and what was going on with me. Our sex life had come to a standstill. I had no sex drive. It could have been because of the 20 milligrams of Paxil that I was taking for my depression. Or it might have been the blood pressure medication, which I took in high doses. Or it could have been plain old fatigue. You don't feel much like having sex when all you want to do is lie down and rest.

What with all of my ailments and the depression and the fatigue, I started to think my life was coming to an end. Family life had become nothing but domestic tasks, and it seemed as though every week my body was failing in another way. I was on medication for depression but it didn't help because I had this sense of impending doom. I wondered what would happen next that would cause me to be put on even more medication. I was unsure and frightened.

One day I was talking with the therapist I saw for my depression, and she mentioned that she had some other clients who'd benefited from going to the compounding pharmacy in Palm Desert and getting natural hormone therapy. I went there, and they recommended I see Dr. Platt. Since I had consulted with at least 25 or 30 doctors, I was a little skeptical about seeing Dr. Platt. But I was desperate.

Soon after I went in for my intake interview, I started the meal plan and I got off caffeine and sugar. A week later I started taking DHEA, progesterone, testosterone, and a T3 thyroid preparation. Dr. Platt told me about the Synthroid I'd been taking for years, which previous doctors had prescribed for my low thyroid. He explained to me that my body was unable to convert Synthroid's T4 into T3, which is the actual thyroid hormone that does all the metabolic work of the thyroid gland. Apparently I'd been taking Synthroid all those years, and it hadn't been doing anything for me.

My energy level increased drastically. Between the hormones, the increase in protein, the diet in general, and the removal of medications that had been throwing my body off balance, I found a big difference in my ability to function.

Once I had more energy, I wasn't as grouchy or impatient as I used to be. I was able to deal with things better both emotionally and physically. The best part has been my ability to participate with my family more. Whereas I used to let my husband take the children out while I stayed home and rested, now I can participate in family outings. Our church has volleyball twice a month, and now I enjoy playing that with my family. We go walking and sightseeing. My children are so happy that mom can go places with them now; I think they feel comfortable that mommy will be there with them.

Also, before, we had no social life as a family. Now we try to have guests visit the house twice a month to eat with us. My husband and I go out with other couples more often. I also see his family more, which I enjoy.

Being able to socialize again, especially with my family, has been so wonderful. For something so simple, it's astonishing.

THE ROOTS OF FATIGUE

Let's talk about fatigue. It came very close to ruining Rhonda's home life. She went to doctor after doctor, and no one could help her. Does that sound familiar? If it does, you're not alone. In my practice I meet many women who go to bed exhausted and wake up tired. They've lost their zest for life, and they feel inadequate to the demands of a normal life.

Rhonda's fatigue was caused by multiple factors, all of them influenced by an imbalance of hormones. The main source of her fatigue was fibromyalgia—again, a very common condition and mostly ignored by the medical community. An important hormone associated with this condition is thyroid. Just getting the thyroid into balance often leads to a reduction in symptoms.

Another cause of her fatigue was recurrent hypoglycemia, which is a low blood sugar or a rapid drop in blood sugar, a condition caused by the over-production of insulin, often due to a lack of progesterone. Any time insulin levels go up, blood sugar goes down. When you take sugar from the brain, the brain gets severely fatigued (many readers will note this happening between 3 and 4 in the afternoon). Progesterone helps to stabilize blood sugar and often eliminates afternoon fatigue.

Another cause of Rhonda's fatigue was depression. This too was caused by a low progesterone level, as well as the internalization of anger. She also had asthma, which can lower oxygen levels in the body, contributing to fatigue.

A low thyroid level by itself can cause fatigue. Furthermore, Rhonda was on Claritin for allergies and Paxil for depression—and the side effects of both drugs include weakness and fatigue.

Why couldn't her doctors help her? As I've said before, doctors are for the most part unaware of the pivotal role of hormones in sustaining health. They simply don't know how easy it is to help people like Rhonda. For me, turning Rhonda's health around was simple: we adjusted a couple of little things here and there. It's not hard to take care of patients. You just have to listen to them and be aware of how hormones affect the body.

Rhonda's brand of fatigue was something I would never have confused with chronic fatigue syndrome, which is a disease associated with fevers and swollen lymph glands. But I think many doctors misdiagnose people like Rhonda, treating them for chronic fatigue syndrome when what they actually have is a simple case of unbalanced hormones. You can see how people like Rhonda could be labeled as having chronic fatigue syndrome. The signs and symptoms are there, but the underlying causes are different.

DRUGS AND MORE DRUGS

This brings up another point I will make again and again in this book: many members of the medical community tend to over-prescribe drugs as a consequence of misdiagnosing simple hormone imbalances. Besides the anti-depressant Paxil, Rhonda was also taking Claritin, prednisone, Prevacid, and Synthroid. Each drug was causing one or more side effects, and Rhonda's body was spiraling out of control under the influence of all of these chemicals.

My first step with patients like Rhonda is to get them off of as many medications as possible while giving them proges-terone to start the healing process. However, with some drugs, such as Paxil, usage should be gradually tapered off, not simply stopped "cold turkey."

Progesterone helps take away asthma, so they can soon start weaning themselves off any asthma medications they might be taking, too. In fact, progesterone has a significantly positive influence on asthma in both men and women. I suspect it is estrogen that creates asthma in many people. Keep in mind that men and women have the same hormones.

A male patient, 57 years old, who came to see me because of weight concerns, was on four medications for asthma. When I told him that in three weeks he would be off all of his asthma medications, he responded, "Doc, I've had asthma for 35 years, and the Mayo Clinic prescribes my medications." I said, "Watch." Three weeks later he came into my office, sat down, and said, "Doc, you won't believe this … I'm off all of my medications for asthma!"

Progesterone treats asthma for two reasons—it blocks estrogen, a very common cause of asthma, and it breaks down into cortisone, which relieves asthma. Also, people who are low in progesterone very commonly have hay fever. Very often, within two weeks of starting progesterone all their hay fever and allergies are gone.

> *Keep in mind that men and women have the same hormones.*

The prednisone Rhonda had been prescribed for her asthma was hurting her more than it was helping her. Prednisone has a lot of side effects. It can cause osteoporosis, cataracts, stomach ulcers, and weight gain.

LOW THYROID

Doctors had prescribed Synthroid for Rhonda's low metabolism, but it actually had little effect. This is something we saw with Brenda J., too: she was taking Synthroid but it wasn't helping her thyroid problem.

Rhonda's under-active thyroid condition was missed due to several factors. Rhonda had a condition called secondary hypothyroidism, which is caused by an insufficient amount of TSH being put out by the pituitary. Her free T3 level was below normal. Her pituitary should have been pouring out TSH to elevate this level, but it wasn't. A doctor looking only at Rhonda's TSH levels would fail to diagnose her condition. Correct thyroid testing would have easily picked this up. Her elevated cholesterol also pointed to a low thyroid.

OTHER BENEFITS OF PROGESTERONE

Rhonda had high blood pressure. About 50 percent of the people with high blood pressure have it because they over-produce insulin. As I've mentioned before, hyperinsulinemia (too much insulin in the bloodstream) is associated with low progesterone levels. Sometimes just reducing patients' insulin levels with progesterone relieves their high blood pressure.

The depression Rhonda experienced was at least partly due to low progesterone. Progesterone is a natural anti-depressant, so women with low progesterone are commonly depressed.

Rhonda was a wonderful candidate for progesterone. It had multiple benefits for her. Just by putting her on progesterone I was able to lower her insulin levels, eliminate her high-blood pressure, help her to begin losing weight, help relieve her depression, and get rid of the asthma.

It's possible that the progesterone helped with her acid reflux problem, too. Rhonda was on a drug called Prevacid, which reduces acid secretion. By lowering insulin levels and reducing certain carbohydrates, you can relieve acid reflux.

SUMMING UP

Getting Rhonda's life turned around was a simple matter of adding several hormones and eliminating the medications she was taking, which removed their concomitant side effects.

In her initial interview, Rhonda indicated she was on a number of medications including thyroid, an antihistamine, an anti-depressant, prednisone, and a medication to prevent acid reflux. Although she was taking thyroid medication, like many people, she was unable to convert the thyroid she was given into the active form, so she remained hypothyroid in spite of being treated. This, of course, contributed to her feeling tired all the time.

Rhonda was estrogen dominant and low in progesterone. This was the cause of her miscarriages, difficulty with conception, morning sickness, fibroid tumors, and endometriosis. Another symptom of low progesterone levels is high insulin levels. Insulin controls blood sugar: when insulin goes up, blood sugar goes down. When the brain doesn't get enough blood sugar, it falls asleep. This, too, contributed to her overall sense of fatigue.

Yet another factor contributing to her fatigue was depression. Some of Rhonda's depression was related to suppressed anger, which manifested as fibromyalgia, a condition in which the body contracts its muscles even during sleep. Patients with this condition wake up stiff in the morning, often in pain, and feeling as though they haven't had enough rest. Prolonged muscle tensing uses up energy, causing daytime fatigue.

Estrogen dominance and low progesterone levels also contributed to Rhonda's developing allergies and asthma. She was placed on antihistamines, which unfortunately compounded her fatigue. The prednisone she was taking for asthma elevates sugar levels. The high blood sugar led to more insulin production, which added to Rhonda's hypoglycemia, a condition that results in feelings of fatigue.

The anti-depressant Paxil has its own list of multiple side effects, including weight gain, loss of libido and—you guessed it—fatigue. When you add up all of the fatigue-inducing chemicals she was both ingesting and producing within her own body, it's a wonder Rhonda was able to accomplish anything at all.

Again, my approach to this patient was simply to deal with the underlying causes rather than the symptoms of her fatigue. Adding progesterone balanced her estrogen dominance and restored her insulin level to normal. This in turn eliminated her asthma, part of her depression, her hypoglycemia, and her allergies, which allowed me to wean her off the fatigue-inducing medications prednisone and Paxil.

At this point we were halfway home. The patient had more control over her life, she was feeling better, and as a result, she was not feeling so angry. Then her fibromyalgia, with all the associated muscle tensing and fatigue, went away. Adding T3, the thyroid hormone her body was craving, gave her even more feelings of well-being, allowing her to lose weight and move even further away from depression.

THE FUEL TO KEEP FAMILIES RUNNING

Rhonda continues to do well with her weight and, more importantly, with her energy and ability to function in her family. I have had other patients who weren't so lucky. I have seen marriages flounder on the issue of fatigue. Without a high energy level it's almost impossible to be effective as a homemaker and mother.

When I read the statistics about the vast number of American women taking anti-depressants, I wonder how many of them would be better served having their metabolisms energized through the use of natural hormones. I would like to see more doctors understand the role hormones play in creating and sustaining a normal zest for life—something that is everyone's birthright.

MIGRAINE HEADACHES
AND KAREN H.

CHAPTER FIVE

Karen is a fashionable woman in her 50s who came to me to solve a post-menopausal weight problem. Her medical history indicated that she'd suffered from migraine headaches all her life. She was amazed when I told her that the migraines were curable. She'd tried to get help with them, spending a considerable amount of money, but to no avail. Readers who have been tolerating migraines should learn from her example: it's never too late to defeat an old enemy like migraines, although the earlier you address this problem the better. I'll let Karen tell you her story:

I've gotten migraine headaches about three or four times a month for my entire life. There would be this intense throbbing behind my right eyeball, in my temples, a neck ache, and nausea. Doctors didn't diagnose these headaches as migraines because I didn't see "auras"— the white light migraine sufferers typically see. I also was not sensitive to light and I did not need to go into a dark room. Only when I was in my 50s, was I told they were migraines.

So when I was young I just called them "my headaches" and took codeine to lessen the pain. When I was 29 years old, I had one so bad that it sent me to the emergency room at the local hospital. I was vomiting, the pain was excruciating, and I thought, "Nobody has headaches like this." I asked my friend to drive me to the emergency room. They treated me with a muscle relaxant and Valium. The next day I just soldiered on and went to work.

The second time I went to the emergency room with a migraine, one of the doctors said it was a severe sinus headache, and he recommended nose surgery. I did have nose surgery and it didn't do a thing.

The third time a migraine sent me to the hospital, the doctors wouldn't let me leave without doing a spinal tap on me. My symptoms were nearly identical to what you see in people who are about to have a stroke, an aneurysm, or who have spinal meningitis. That gives you an idea of how severe the migraines were.

I was told the headaches might go away after menopause, but they didn't. When menopause failed to give me relief, I finally went to see a neurosurgeon. My headaches were diagnosed as migraines and I was given two medications that finally helped. He gave me Inderal and Imitrex. The Inderal reduced the frequency of the headaches to once every six weeks or so, which was a blessing. Whenever I did feel a headache coming on, I would self-inject the Imitrex, which would stop the progression and leave me without pain.

Naturally, I was grateful for this relief after all those years of suffering. But I would later find out that Inderal and Imitrex were just masking the pain, not getting to the cause of it.

Meanwhile, I stopped smoking. The combination of stopping smoking and going through menopause caused me to gain 50 pounds. This was scary to me. I had always been pretty close to the weight I wanted to be. I was one of those Twiggy-generation people who was always trying to lose 10 pounds—you can never be quite thin enough— but, generally speaking, I didn't have a weight problem. But once I had gained the 50 pounds I was scared. I looked matronly, felt old, and I didn't know whether I would ever be able to lose this weight.

I heard a friend talking about Dr. Platt, and she spoke so highly of him that I decided to go to him for weight loss.

I went to see him and we talked for an hour. I was comfortable with him, and I was fascinated that he's a traditionally trained M.D. who has a philosophy that crosses over into alternative medicine. He told me he could eliminate my migraine headaches and that losing the 50 pounds would be just the icing on the cake.

He put me on progesterone, thyroid medication, and DHEA and started weaning me off the Inderal as well as the HRT my gynecologist had put me on at menopause.

At some point during the weaning from Inderal I had a terrible, terrible night when I couldn't put my head on a pillow because my head hurt so much. It wasn't like a migraine; it was like every one of my hairs hurt my scalp. If I touched my hair, my scalp was in agony. I spent the night sitting up, catching whatever sleep I could, and the next morning I called Dr. Platt's office and went to see him.

He told me what was happening—that I was getting my nerve endings back. The drugs I'd been taking had numbed them, and now they were coming back to life. He told me the symptoms would be gone within 36 hours, and he was right. It is now 20 months since I first saw Dr. Platt, and I have not had a single migraine headache.

It was also the easiest weight loss I have ever experienced. I stuck to the diet religiously and the pounds just melted off. I lost eight pounds the first week and about three pounds every successive week. I started in September and by Thanksgiving I had lost 32 pounds. I felt great, I wasn't hungry, and I wasn't getting headaches! At Thanksgiving I went off the diet because I had tons of guests and relatives coming in for the holidays, and my passion is cooking for people. But I plan to go back on the diet at some point to lose the last 18 pounds.

The weight I lost was a different kind of 32 pounds—I can't quite explain it, but I had this feeling that I was losing stored-up fat from a long time ago. There is a different definition to my body. It looks and feels different.

The other day I was cleaning out my medicine cabinet and I came upon some Imitrex shots that were still good. One part of me wanted to keep them—what if I got another headache? These things were lifesavers at one point in my life. But I had the courage to throw them out. I've been headache-free for 20 months, through all kinds of changes in my diet, and I don't see any reason why that should change.

PROGESTERONE AND MIGRAINES

Karen is another example of a woman who had been estrogen dominant her entire life. Migraine headaches are one result of the adverse effect estrogen has on blood vessels.

You might ask, why did Karen feel the toxicity of estrogen as migraines, while in someone like Brenda J. it took the form of fibroid tumors and troubled pregnancies? As I've explained before, there are receptor sites for hormones all over the body, and in different people different sites predominate. Thus the symptoms of estrogen dominance will vary according to where a person's estrogen sites are located. I suppose one could say that Karen was lucky her excess estrogen didn't eventually cause breast or ovarian cancer. However, you'd have had a hard time convincing Karen of her good luck in the middle of a migraine attack. Those are brutal. I once treated a woman who had severe menstrual migraines starting at age 14 with her first menses. On two occasions she had paralytic migraines resulting in strokes.

Everyone knows somebody who has migraines, and everyone knows how excruciating they are, so it's quite remarkable that the medical community has missed the simple fact that natural progesterone is a cost-effective cure for menstrual migraines. There are millions of women out there like Karen all desperate for relief. Many of them attend pain clinics and explore every avenue they can—meditation, acupressure, and so on—but continue to suffer month after month.

Karen went all the way from her teenage years—when her body first started producing estrogen—to menopause suffering from these headaches. At menopause, she might have hoped to get some relief since her body was reducing its production of estrogen, but doctors placed her on hormone replacement therapy (HRT), which made sure the migraines continued.

All she needed to solve a lifelong problem was progesterone, the hormone that protects women from the effects of too much estrogen. As long as she continues taking it, Karen won't have any more migraine headaches.

She also tested low in thyroid, which isn't surprising in someone with low progesterone levels, because progesterone has a major influence on the thyroid. Giving her the right thyroid medication helped her to lose weight in a comfortable fashion.

When Karen talks about feeling as though she was losing stored-up fat and seeing her body change in a way she had not seen before, she is talking about the difference between a fat-burning weight loss program and a muscle-burning calorie restriction diet. In her youth, Karen did a lot of calorie restriction diets—those grapefruit-and-lean-meat diets that were popular in the 1960s and 1970s. Those make you lose muscle. They give you a sagging look, make your skin look droopy, and impair muscle tone. To Karen, actually losing fat and seeing some muscle definition was a revelation.

Would it be fair to say that Karen felt eliminating her migraine headaches with a natural bio-identical hormone was a miracle?

POSTPARTUM DEPRESSION AND SUSAN B.

CHAPTER SIX

When I first started to write this book, the headlines were filled with news of the trial of Andrea Yates, the woman who struggled with postpartum depression and eventually drowned her five children. Although I think Yates' problems went well beyond postpartum depression, it was a major factor in her breakdown. This is a very real condition that causes untold misery to new mothers. Fortunately, it is easy to treat.

Susan B. found a solution to her postpartum depression by balancing her hormones. I hope her experience will be instructive to other mothers, particularly breastfeeding mothers, who can avoid the side effects of psychogenic drugs by taking this approach. I'll let Susan tell you what happened:

Depression has been a problem in my family for a long time. My mother and sister and I seemed always to be depressed when I was growing up. Eventually my mother committed suicide, when I was 16 years old.

Along with our depression went low metabolism, and, in my case, I can't remember when I wasn't battling my weight. I ate normal amounts of food but I was always fat.

Once, as an adult, I got so fed up with always being fat that I went on this rigorous program, exercising three hours a day, six days a week. I did slim down, of course. But it was impossible to keep up that kind of schedule. As soon as I slacked off even a little bit, the weight came right back on.

At the age of 45 I had a child. The moment she was born, I went into a massive depression. It was difficult caring for the baby because I didn't feel any of the joy of motherhood but I still had all of the daily responsibilities. One day I was talking to my doctor about my depression, complaining a bit about how being over-weight contributed to my overall feelings of hopelessness. She told me about other patients of hers who had taken off weight by going to Dr. Platt. I decided to go see him, figuring that slimming down would be one way of improving my situation. Little did I realize it would be the solution to my depression, too.

I was a size 20 when I went to see him. I weighed 190 pounds—it was hard just moving around with that much weight on my 5'3" frame. At first I just went on the diet and held off taking the hormones he had recommended. After a few months I lost 22 pounds.

At that point Dr. Platt said I had to start progesterone and thyroid. So he started me on both of those and, my God, what a difference it made in my mood! It was an incredible difference. I feel like I'm a different person today, like a person I haven't seen in about 10 years.

Two months after starting the hormones I was able to start weaning myself off my prescription anti-depressants.

With the progesterone and the thyroid medication, I had lots of energy and a whole new outlook on life. The other beneficial thing was what it did for my skin. My skin looked so much better after I started the progesterone. It became more radiant, which is a great thing to have happen at my age. I used to have all of these skin tags on my neck, and about a month after I started the progesterone they all disappeared.

Ultimately, it took me ten months to lose about 60 pounds and get down to a size 4. I must have gained a lot of muscle mass, because I don't weigh 105 pounds like most size 4 women. I weigh 137 pounds. Of course, with more muscle mass my metabolism is much higher than it used to be, so it is that much easier to maintain my weight while still eating the foods I love to eat.

A LIFETIME OF BATTLING OBESITY

Susan B. is typical of the many people who have fought obesity their entire life not because of an eating problem but because of a hormone problem.

> *I believe the only cause for postpartum depression is low progesterone.*

Susan had the classic history of someone with a low progesterone level who becomes estrogen dominant and depressed. I believe the only cause for postpartum depression is low progesterone. In the second and third trimesters the placenta pours out progesterone, which is why women feel so good during this time of their pregnancy. But after the baby is delivered, progesterone levels go down.

For most women, once they start ovulating again, their bodies begin producing progesterone and their moods lift. But Susan was low in progesterone to begin with, and she was in her 40s, when hormone levels are on the decline anyway. So she had no source of progesterone.

Her low progesterone caused high insulin levels—the number one cause of obesity. Low progesterone also led to an increase in estrogen—another hormone that creates fat. Low progesterone leads to depression and other psychological problems.

She also had the standard symptoms of an under-active thyroid: her skin was dry, her nails didn't grow well, she was easily fatigued, and so on. Her blood tests bore out this deficiency. Her low thyroid contributed to her depression, too. The thyroid has a tremendous influence on the metabolism of every cell of the body, including the brain cells.

Helping Susan was a very simple matter. As soon as her hormones were balanced she regained a zest for living. The weight loss made her feel even better—it was a particularly sweet reward for a woman who had spent half a lifetime struggling with obesity.

I hope you, the reader, are beginning to understand the importance of hormones when it comes to health. Susan's case is another example of a deficiency of hormones creating havoc with one's health and illustrates the importance of being pro-active with your own health care. For the most part, you cannot expect the medical community to come up with answers it is ill-equipped to find.

EVEN MOVIE STARS GET THE BLUES

As many of you are aware, actress/model Brooke Shields wrote a book detailing her experience with severe postpartum depression. Her advice to women with this problem is to avail themselves of anti-depressant medications. She has been on multiple talk shows reiterating this advice.

What she is proposing is the classic, standard medical care approach: take a Band-Aid (drug) for your problem.

It is my understanding that Ms. Shields utilized in vitro fertilization to get pregnant. The number one reason why a woman cannot get pregnant is a low progesterone level. My understanding is that she did not have morning sickness, the occurrence of which I would have expected. After her delivery, her progesterone level might have dropped to non-existent levels, which could have precipitated her severe postpartum depression.

Using natural, bio-identical progesterone might have eliminated the need for in vitro fertilization and prevented postpartum depression. In fact, giving her progesterone would have eliminated her depression almost immediately.

There is an ironic twist to this situation. Many of you might be aware that actor Tom Cruise, who I understand is a practicing Scientologist, advised Ms. Shields to take a more natural approach for her depression—healing with prayer, and so on.

Interestingly, Tom Cruise has said that he has a problem with ADHD—a condition I feel is also caused by a low progesterone level. So both of these well-known actors have the same hormone deficiency, in my view, yet neither of them is aware of it.

FIBROMYALGIA AND JANET L.

CHAPTER SEVEN

Fibromyalgia is a rheumatism of the muscles, ligaments, and tendons that can cause crippling pain and can make normal activity excruciating. It is far more common than most people realize and seems to occur with great frequency among overweight people. Fibromyalgia can be healed using a natural, drugless approach, a fact that should bring joy to the hearts of many sufferers. I hope Janet's story will inspire others to "say no" to this debilitating condition and begin living a pain-free, joyous life.

I've had fibromyalgia for 20 years, although it wasn't diagnosed until recently. Most people who have fibromyalgia do not get properly diagnosed until they have had it for at least seven years. That's because it is a progressive disease, and when it starts out it might only manifest as a stiff neck or isolated pain and general fatigue. The symptoms, in other words, are so general they can be interpreted as the flu, tired muscles, a sleep disorder, or any number of less serious problems.

When I first started experiencing the pain of fibromyalgia I was living in the mountains in Washington State. In that often cold, usually moist climate my body behaved like a barometer—

whenever the weather changed my body would feel it. Whether it was dampness, cold, a change in the wind—any change would register in my body as pain. I went to rheumatologists, chiropractors, all kinds of doctors about my pain, but none of them had a solution for me.

One doctor started me on cortisone shots. We reached a point where he was shooting cortisone into 42 muscles in my back every day. He finally said, "Janet, I can't do this any more. You've become a human pincushion."

I would have good days and bad days. On my good days I was energetic and took part in family activities with great zest. On bad days I wouldn't be able to get dressed without stopping a few times to lie down and rest and get my energy back.

In the days before the fibromyalgia was advanced, my husband and I decided to build our dream house up in the mountains in Cardiff. I took a very active part in designing it, a house on three levels. It was a project that went on for several years. By the time we were close to finishing it, the major symptoms of my fibromyalgia had set in. At that point, I found it unbearable to climb stairs. I had to wonder who that person was who had thought to design a three-story house. But no one had diagnosed me or told me my problem would get worse every year.

I was given various medications for pain, Neurontin being the one I ended up taking long-term. It dulled the pain without getting at the source of the problem.

The way I dealt with the pain in the early days was to be very active. Inactivity seemed to exacerbate the stiffness and pain, so I threw myself into family activities. We have a large extended family up north and I loved making dinners and entertaining. I could forget about my pain if I had a goal like cooking for 40 people. However, the activity took a lot out of me and after these dinners were over I would have to recuperate for a week.

Part of the fibromyalgia was a sleeping problem—the pain kept me awake. Often I would get only three hours of sleep at night. I would toss and turn and then finally go to my husband's recliner to get some sleep. It was easier to find a comfortable position there. I also started getting migraine headaches.

Gradually I reached the point where I was quite debilitated. If it were snowing outside I could only walk a half a block or so before exhaustion would set in. My knees would get so swollen they would be like footballs. I couldn't bend them.

A rheumatologist finally diagnosed me. He checked my pressure points and told me all 18 of them were inflamed. He said I had both osteoarthritis and fibromyalgia.

I finally had a diagnosis, but the rheumatologist didn't have a solution for my pain. He just prescribed more Neurontin. My husband and I arrived at the point where we were ready to sacrifice our dream house so we could live in a warm, dry climate where I could be in less pain. We sold our house in Cardiff and bought a house in the desert. As soon as we'd moved in I contacted a rheumatologist—I needed a local source for my Neurontin. This doctor checked my pressure points, and they were, as usual, inflamed.

Meanwhile, I happened to see Dr. Platt on television talking about hormones and weight loss. I thought that if I could lose some weight I might be able to move around better. I weighed 185 back then, and I am 5 feet tall. The weight seemed to exacerbate my pain. So I decided to go in to see him.

He was astounding. I sat and talked to him for two and a half hours for my first visit! He went over all my records, and then he started asking me such pointed questions that I kept on saying to myself, "How did he know that?"

He told me I was internalizing anger and that I needed to face what was angering me and cope with it. We talked about some fairly personal stuff. He gave me some ideas for changing the patterns in my life that were forcing me to swallow all this anger. He said I could put the fibromyalgia into remission through lifestyle changes and balancing my hormones.

I started taking progesterone and I went on the diet. Three weeks after seeing Dr. Platt I went to see the rheumatologist. He checked my pressure points and told me there was no more inflammation. I told him that for the first time I was able to sleep through the night and that I didn't have pain any more. This was three weeks after starting the progesterone! The rheumatologist said, "Whatever you're doing, continue doing it. Your osteoarthritis has gone into remission."

I got really excited about how effective the progesterone had been. The next time I went in to see Dr. Platt I wanted to have a whole blood panel done. If one hormone could take away all that pain, what else could we accomplish by balancing all of my hormones?

When he examined my blood panel, Dr. Platt said that I had a thyroid deficiency. He gave me a prescription for thyroid medication and my energy level increased dramatically. I continued with the diet, eventually losing 53 pounds. Today I weigh 132 and I feel so incredible, it's as though someone gave me back my life from years ago. I feel young inside. When I visited my grandchildren up north last time, I went hiking and swimming with them, things I'd never been able to do. "It's like we have a new grandma!" all the kids said.

Dr. Platt also prescribed testosterone, which has given me back my sex life—my husband is absolutely thrilled.

I feel so blessed to have met Dr. Platt. He's changed my life. Some of my friends ask me whether I'd have sold my dream house if I'd known I was going to feel this good—today I'd have no problem with those flights of stairs. But I know everything happens for a reason. I'm just grateful things have turned out the way they have.

AN UNDER-RECOGNIZED DISEASE

Janet's long and unsuccessful quest to get help with her fibromyalgia doesn't surprise me at all. Only about 50 percent of doctors even acknowledge the reality of the disease. Even if they make the diagnosis, they usually tell their patients there's no known cure. The reason the majority of doctors say they cannot cure fibromyalgia is because they are unaware of its probable causes.

In my experience, a large part of the cause is internalization of anger. The other major cause is an imbalance in hormones.

Every patient I've ever treated for fibromyalgia has been someone who internalizes anger. Often they are perfectionists who have unrealistically high expectations of themselves and of the people living around them. They allow the behavior of other people to control how they feel or allow the world they deal with to make them angry. From what I have seen with my patients, the challenge for those with fibromyalgia is often this issue of control. This means disappointments can be many.

Think of a person with "road rage"; he or she is allowing other drivers to determine how they feel. Instead of road rage, fibromyalgia sufferers have "life-in-general rage."

The response to loss of control is anger, which they often do not realize is internalized. The anger causes, in turn, a general tensing of muscles. When muscles are tensed, two things happen: lactic acid builds up, causing pain (athletes call it muscle burn), and a large amount of energy is expended, causing persistent fatigue.

At night the mind may continue to deal with something that is frustrating, so all night long their muscles tense. The jaw tightens, causing them to grind their teeth or develop TMJ (temporomandibular joint dysfunction). A lot of anger could also be internalized into the GI tract, causing problems with constipation and diarrhea, often referred to as IBS (irritable bowel syndrome). People with fibromyalgia often awaken in the morning with aches and pains: upper back pain, neck pain, low back pain, and pain along the sides of the hips.

Fibromyalgia sufferers are often people who can't say no. They wind up having unwanted house guests, having Thanksgiving and Christmas dinners at their house every year (talk about stress!), taking care of aging parents, and so on.

Very often they live with a controlling mate. They continually walk around "on eggshells," with their muscles perpetually tensed whether they are aware of it or not, always trying to please their mate.

Another common example of anger due to loss of control is the patient who can't lose weight. They are dieting, exercising, cutting out fat, doing everything they think is right, and they cannot lose an ounce. Imagine their anger when they look in the mirror every day. Their inability to lose weight is controlling them.

Part of my approach with fibromyalgia patients is to give them insight into their anger and work with them to discover ways to dissipate it. I urge them to make changes in their lives and to seek the help of a therapist, if necessary, to deal with the source of their anger. I explain to my patients that I can get their hormones into balance, but I cannot eliminate their anger. However, I help them begin to deal with the sources of negative energy in their lives.

FIBROMYALGIA AND METABOLISM

Janet L. and I had discussions about her anger, and she started taking steps to change certain parts of her life accordingly. Meanwhile, I explained that her under-active thyroid was contributing to her problem. The thyroid gland has a tremendous influence on muscle tissue, and when you're dealing with fibromyalgia, you're dealing with muscle tissue. The condition that causes the greatest damage to the muscles—more than heart attacks, more than anything else—is an under-active thyroid. Every patient I've ever treated for fibromyalgia has had an under-active thyroid.

For muscles to work properly, one must replace certain fuels they require that may have been depleted. The major fuels include d-ribose, coenzyme Q-10, and magnesium—all available in health food stores.

I put Janet on thyroid medication and replaced certain supplements, and that was the beginning of a healing process for her muscles that eventually left her pain-free. I also prescribed progesterone. It's a feel-good hormone that is effective for everyone, especially women.

Janet responded nicely to the hormones, to the weight loss, and most especially to getting rid of her anger. Today she's a very happy woman.

THE MISSING LINK

So far I have talked about one aspect of fibromyalgia—the internalization of anger and the associated muscle tension, causing the buildup of lactic acid and fatigue. Now I'd like to identify what I feel is another very common underlying cause of fibromyalgia: ADHD. I do not make this statement lightly. It is based on years of treating patients with adult ADHD. ADHD is associated with high levels of adrenaline, the fight-or-flight hormone. This can cause an increase in anger, stress, nervous tension, or rage. Any of these emotions can cause muscle tension, leading to a buildup of lactic acid and subsequently fibromyalgia. Very often, getting rid of the excess adrenaline goes a long way toward eliminating fibromyalgia.

WHEN ALL ELSE FAILS

A number of my patients have had the perfect psychological and physiological characteristics for fibromyalgia—yet they experienced no muscle tenderness. The one characteristic these people invariably shared was that they practiced breathing exercises. Nothing that I am aware of brings about better muscle relaxation than deep breathing.

With eyes closed, take in a deep breath in slowly, hold it for a few seconds, then let it out slowly. Try to keep the mind blank. Doing this for a few minutes several times a day can be extremely beneficial. Taking a deep breath when you feel anger coming on can help relieve muscle tension.

Deep breathing provides a dual benefit—it relaxes muscles directly and, at the same time, enhances the flow of lymph. The body's lymph system helps to drain waste products, which includes lactic acid, from muscle tissues.

The secret to a long life is to keep on breathing.

Every moment that you spend upset, in despair, in anguish, angry or hurt because of the behavior of anybody else in your life is a moment in which you have given up control of your life.

— WAYNE DYER

OSTEOPOROSIS—MYTH VERSUS REALITY

CHAPTER EIGHT

Not too long ago, osteoporosis was associated with fractured hips and often led to permanent residence in a nursing home. Nowadays, the scenario is about the same, except that, because of modern surgical methods, nursing homes are rarely the patient's final destination any more.

With the advent of DEXA scans, which measure bone density, we can now measure the state of bone health and easily measure the extent, if any, of bone loss. These studies can also be used to assess the response (if any) to therapy. DEXA stands for dual-energy X-ray absorptionmetry. The most important measurement is called the T-score, a measure of the standard deviation away from the "norm," which is based on the bone density in a 24-year-old person. A reading of -2.5 below the norm is considered osteoporosis. A reading between -1.0 and -2.5 is designated as osteopenia.

The diagnosis "osteopenia" was created after DEXA scans were put in use. Realistically, a person in their 50s or 60s is not likely to have the same bone density as a person in their mid 20s. So is this a condition that needs pharmaceutical intervention, or if it a natural condition of aging that simply requires hormonal balance and natural supplementation to maintain bone health? This question is important because doctors often prescribe the same toxic medications for osteopenia as they do for osteoporosis.

Again, this book is not intended as a diatribe against conventional medicine. However, I feel patients should be better informed so that perhaps more healthful decisions can be made.

TRADITIONAL TREATMENTS FOR OSTEOPOROSIS AND OSTEOPENIA

The traditional approach to treating osteoporosis in women was to give them estrogen, usually in the form of Premarin, along with a high dose of calcium. Improving bone health was touted as one of the major benefits of taking estrogen. The problem is, there has never been a single study indicating that estrogen has any benefit in reversing osteoporosis—in fact, in 1999 the FDA eliminated osteoporosis as an indication for giving estrogen. It is true that when a woman is still having menstrual cycles, and for several years after menopause, estrogen does have a positive effect on bone health. But it will not prevent the eventual onset of osteoporosis.

The main classes of therapeutic drugs utilized for osteoporosis (and, unfortunately, osteopenia) are called bisphosphonates. They go by several brand names, such as Fosamax, Actonel, and Binova. Bone is in a constant state of regeneration, aided by cells that help resorb bone (the osteoclasts), and then cells that build bone (the osteoblasts). The bisphosphonates act in a way that prevents the osteoclasts from resorbing bone but at the same time prevents the osteoblasts from forming new bone.

As a result, you wind up with old, brittle bone that looks good on a DEXA scan but can actually be more easily fractured than an untreated bone. This is certainly not the desired effect.

In addition, bisphosphonates have serious potential side effects. They are very similar to the same chemicals used to clear drain pipes and clean away bathtub residue. This is why it is necessary to avoid lying down after taking these pills because they can eat a hole through the esophagus. They can also cause gastric erosions and severe diarrhea.

Other side effects include blindness and a condition referred to as osteonecrosis—an eating away of the jaw bone leading to the teeth falling out as well as other dental nightmares.

Bisphosphonates are the largest-selling drugs in the world for osteoporosis and, unfortunately, osteopenia as well. Another fact to keep in mind is that these drugs have a ten-year half-life, which means this is how long it takes to eliminate 50 percent of the medication from your body.

So what about taking calcium supplements—another traditional approach that no one seems to question? Is it really safe and is it necessary?

Consider the fact that most of the foods we eat have calcium in their makeup. In 35 years of practice, I have never seen a patient with a calcium deficiency. Interestingly enough, Asians, who traditionally cannot digest milk products due to a low level of lactase, have an extremely low incidence of osteoporosis.

Another thing to consider: Is it possible that taking an excess of calcium may enhance calcification (hardening) of our arteries? Doctors actually use calcium channel blocking agents to treat coronary artery disease and lower blood pressure. Calcium stimulates gastric acid secretion, which possibly contributes to reflux esophagitis. There are other concerns as well. Calcium can promote prostate cancer and can also promote kidney stones.

My own feeling is that if one does take calcium, perhaps in the form of calcium citrate, it is wise to limit the intake to one tablet per day. Magnesium is a lot more important than calcium for building bones and should be taken in a quantity two to three times that of calcium.

A BETTER APPROACH TO BONE HEALTH

There are two points of view to consider with osteoporosis and osteopenia—prevention and treatment. Since this book is about hormones, and since hormones are important for both prevention and treatment, let us start with them.

> *I, for one, suspect that the number one cause of osteoporosis in both men and women is a low progesterone level.*

The primary hormones involved in bone health are testosterone, progesterone, estrogen, and dihydroepiandosterone, or DHEA. There is a strong hereditary factor to osteoporosis, but what we're really talking about is inheriting a hormonal predisposition to osteoporosis. If a person is aware that their mother or father has or had osteoporosis, then the primary concern should be hormone balance. I, for one, suspect that the number one cause of osteoporosis in both men and women is a low progesterone level.

Women who are on birth control pills, and thereby are not ovulating and have no progesterone, are certainly setting themselves up for bone problems. On the other hand, women who are estrogen dominant (who have or did have PMS, cramps, breast tenderness, and so on) often have great bone densities; however, they also have a high incidence of breast cancer. Balance seems to be the key when it comes to estrogen.

Testosterone is also intricately involved with bone metabolism. Women who have had hysterectomies, whether total (with the ovaries removed) or partial (with the ovaries left in) will have low testosterone levels. In men, the level of testosterone starts dropping when they are in their 20s and continues steadily downward. A man who has lost his libido, often due to low testosterone, is a person obviously at risk for osteoporosis.

Osteoporosis in men, the incidence of which is almost on a par with women, can have deadly consequences. A fractured hip in a male over the age of 65 is associated with a 25 percent mortality rate during the following year. In addition, men very commonly have low progesterone levels. This situation becomes moot around the age of 50 when virtually all men stop producing progesterone.

Needless to say, I feel that both testosterone and progesterone are extremely important for preventing osteoporosis. DHEA is another hormone that gradually but consistently declines as we age; it is a balancing hormone, in that it helps produce both estrogen and testosterone—both being important for bone health.

ADDITIONAL CONSIDERATIONS

Another hormone that certainly bears mentioning is melatonin, which is put out by the pineal gland. It is generally known as the hormone that puts us to sleep at night. However, it has other functions as well. It is extremely important in bone metabolism. It also plays a significant role with regard to our immune system. It helps to produce natural killer cells and interleukin-2, both of which the body uses to fight cancer on a daily basis (cells are constantly mutating and have to be dealt with regularly). The problem is that we stop producing this hormone around the age of 60. So one should consider melatonin for both prevention and treatment of osteoporosis, especially as one gets older.

The bottom line concerning osteoporosis is that it can often be prevented—though unfortunately, we live in a world where preventive medicine is not practiced. The preventive approach for osteoporosis is not only a matter of achieving hormonal balance, but includes other factors of extreme importance, such as exercise, proper nutrition, and lack of stress.

I certainly appreciate and admire people who are able to avail themselves of the benefits of a disciplined lifestyle. I am talking about people who eat right, exercise three to four times a week, do breathing exercises to reduce stress, avoid taking medications with toxic side effects, and so on. I know there are millions of people in this category. Not surprisingly, they rarely come to see me. In a perfect world, everyone would live this way—and would maintain a balance of their hormones.

I would recommend, for those who for whatever reason cannot fit precisely into this scheme, a minimum of getting their hormones balanced and utilizing one particular supplement, vitamin D.

VITAMIN D—THE ULTIMATE SUPPLEMENT

First off, vitamin D is not a vitamin. It is considered a prohormone—a substance that converts into a hormone. This helps to explain the multiplicity of its benefits. It is known to help prevent 26 cancers, including cancer of the breast, colon, prostate, and pancreas. Not only does it help prevent cancer, it actually kills cancer cells. It is kind of ironic when you consider that doctors continually advise patients to avoid the sun to prevent skin cancers, which for the most part are readily treatable. Yet for most people the sun is the main source of vitamin D, a substance that helps prevent many types of cancer that are much more dangerous than skin cancers. (By the way, I do not believe melanomas are always sun-related.)

Among its many benefits, vitamin D acts as an ace-inhibitor and may lower blood pressure. In addition, it is reported to effectively prevent the flu, help prevent multiple sclerosis, alleviate seasonal affective disorder, and help prevent Alzheimer's disease.

When it comes to bone health, vitamin D is unsurpassed. In England, where osteoporosis is common because of a lack of sunshine, this condition is often treated only with high dosages of vitamin D. Vitamin D aids in the absorption of calcium from the diet and the deposition of calcium into bone.

My recommendation for the treatment of osteoporosis is 10,000 I.U./day of vitamin D3. Compare this dosage to the RDA (recommended daily allowance) of 200 I.U., which is only enough to prevent rickets, with no other benefit. Most people take 400 to 600 I.U., which I feel is very inadequate to help with osteoporosis. I recommend 5,000 I.U. of vitamin D3 daily as a preventive dose.

BONE-BUILDING SUPPLEMENTS

Vitamin K is extremely important for treating osteoporosis. It takes calcium out of blood vessels and puts it into bone—a double benefit. My recommendation is 10,000 mcg of vitamin K1/K2 daily.

Magnesium, again, is extremely important—much more so than calcium. I recommend taking around 1,000 mg per day.

Strontium is probably the best mineral for building bone.

Other bone-building supplements are boron, whey protein, proline, silica, lycopene, and glutathione (from N-acetyl cysteine and/or alpha lipoic acid), and there are many others.

END THOUGHTS

Every system in the body is controlled by hormones and that includes the skeletal system. Prevention and treatment of osteoporosis requires the use of bio-identical hormone therapy. Taking certain supplements enhances the effect of these hormones, and exercise is the icing on the cake. Together these approaches may help obviate the need for toxic medications, which may not provide the benefits one is looking for in any case.

DHEA—KEY TO WELL-BEING

CHAPTER NINE

One hormone I've given only passing mention to so far is dihydroepiandosterone, or DHEA. All of the effects of this very important hormone have not yet been plumbed by medical science, but we know enough about it to know it is absolutely essential for optimal health.

Since the 1980s many research papers have been published on the multiple healthful functions DHEA performs in the body. It seems to help prevent heart disease, osteoporosis, prostate cancer in men, and breast cancer in women.

DHEA is produced mainly by the adrenal glands, but also by the gonads, the brain, and the skin. At one stage of life—during the teenage years—it is the most abundant steroid hormone in the body. DHEA levels decline in a straight line as we age. This hormone begins to appear in our bodies at age 6, peaks during our 20s, is at the 50 percent level at age 40, and between the ages of 60 and 80 declines to between 20 and 10 percent of peak levels. This definitive decrease is not seen with other hormones, and because of it, DHEA is considered the biological marker for aging: those people with the highest levels seem to have the greatest longevity. In fact, some believe that many of the manifestations of aging are caused by deficiencies in DHEA.

WHAT TO EXPECT

Administration of DHEA is associated with a remarkable increase in perceived physical and psychological well-being. These benefits are noticed after about four months of therapy. People report increased energy, better sleep, a significant improvement in sexuality and in mood, along with a better ability to handle stress.

DHEA has been shown to enhance memory and mental acuity and to decrease depression. Administration of DHEA helps to boost the immune system, improves chronic fatigue syndrome, helps to reduce body fat, and helps address auto-immune diseases such as lupus, ulcerative colitis, and rheumatoid arthritis.

DHEA has its own receptor sites. It raises growth hormone levels and breaks down into testosterone, which may possibly be the reason for some of its benefits.

People with high levels of DHEA have lower incidences of Alzheimer's and Parkinson's disease. Some consider a low DHEA level to be the most significant biological marker for breast cancer in premenopausal women.

When measuring DHEA levels, the proper lab test is the one that assesses DHEA-S, not DHEA.

In men, estradiol levels should be monitored while taking DHEA. Ideally, the estradiol level should not be higher than 20. If it is higher than this to begin with, I do not prescribe DHEA. If the level goes over 40 while the person is on DHEA, I cut back the dosage or the frequency of administration.

When levels of estrogen or testosterone are problematic, another approach is to use a different form of DHEA called 7-keto DHEA. This formulation does not convert into estrogen or testosterone. It can be obtained over the counter; the dosage is 100 mg per day.

DHEA AND STRESS

People who live with a lot of stress start to show lowered DHEA levels after a certain amount of time. Their adrenal glands become exhausted, and since the adrenal glands produce the majority of DHEA, their DHEA levels go way down. Airline pilots, for instance, whose days consist of meeting strict schedules despite unpredictable weather, performing numerous take-offs and landings (landings often involve split-second timing and near misses), and other stressful situations, often show up in my office with little or no DHEA on their hormone panels.

It's well known that pilots report unusually high levels of prostate cancer. Many of them theorize that this might be caused by the radiation they are constantly exposed to, flying at high altitudes. But it's my theory that lack of DHEA may contribute to the problem. Another likely cause is lack of progesterone.

Progesterone, like DHEA, diminishes in people who live under constant stress. The most dramatic example is seen in women living in abusive situations. They very often show almost no DHEA on their hormone panels, and they tend to have all the signs of estrogen dominance as well. Living in constant fear depletes both DHEA and progesterone.

MENOPAUSE AND PERIMENOPAUSE

CHAPTER TEN

I purposefully did not put this chapter at the beginning of the book, even though, for many readers, it will be the most important. Having read through the preceding chapters, you should now have a feel for the importance of hormones—how necessary it is for them to be in balance, and the devastating consequences that occur when they are out of balance. You should also be aware by now of the tragic lack of knowledge among doctors regarding how the body operates with regard to hormones. It is no wonder, then, that the way of treating menopause in women (and andropause in men, which I discuss in chapter 12) has remained basically unchanged for the last 50 years.

This situation has had more consequence for patients than the inconvenience of putting up with symptoms; it has literally put their health at risk for serious diseases and higher death rates. This is particularly the case in two areas where information is deficient: how natural hormones can prevent many of the diseases of aging, and how the incorrect use of hormones can cause unnecessary deaths due to cancer, heart disease, and strokes.

USING BIO-IDENTICAL HORMONES

Perhaps the most commonly known application of hormone therapy is the treatment of women going through menopause. The term "menopause" means the absence of periods, whether the absence occurs naturally or is surgically induced (e.g., due to a hysterectomy).

As women approach the time of menopause, that is, during perimenopause, there is a drop in levels of the hormones produced by the ovaries. This causes a number of symptoms, the most common of which is the onset of irregular periods, which may start occurring sporadically and be of shorter than usual duration. This reflects a drop in estrogen levels. At the same time, a drop in progesterone levels may cause women to experience an increase in PMS (premenstrual syndrome) or cramps, a drop in libido, an increase in weight, and more difficulty in thinking.

Eventually, estrogen and progesterone levels will fall to a level where they can no longer prepare the uterus for bleeding— menopause has begun.

Some women go through this phase of their lives with few or no symptoms. Other women develop hot flashes, night sweats, and other symptoms and become very uncomfortable.

But no matter how you look at it, menopause is a very natural condition that all women eventually go through. The problem is that the medical system has taken this natural condition and turned it into a disease that has to be treated.

Back in the 1960s, Robert Wilson, M.D., a gynecologist in New York City, published a book called *Feminine Forever,* in which he said that when women go through menopause, "they enter a 'vapid cow-like state' and became very unpleasant companions for their husbands." He evidently felt women should be treated for their husbands benefit, not for their own.

He received tremendous financial backing from the makers of Premarin, who helped publish his book and sent him on a nation-wide tour so he could promote Premarin to other physicians around the country.

THE CONTROVERSY OVER PREMARIN

Let me say a few words about Premarin. The name of this manufactured estrogen compound actually delineates its source: pregnant mares' urine. There are about 100 molecules of estrogen in this preparation, but only one of them is similar to a human estrogen. Although it is considered a "natural" hormone since it is derived from a natural substance, clearly it is natural only for horses.

Premarin became the largest-selling drug in the world. However, eventually a darker side to hormone replacement therapy emerged. It is estimated that in the first ten years after the manufacturer started the Premarin market campaign, somewhere between 200,000 and 2,000,000 women developed cancer of the uterus. However, instead of removing Premarin from the market, the drug company added Provera to it. Although this synthetic progesterone reduced the risk of uterine cancer, it quadrupled a woman's chances of getting breast cancer from the estrogen.

Along the way, the drug company started ascribing certain benefits to estrogen replacement therapy without the means to back up their claims.

They claimed that estrogen was beneficial for women with osteoporosis, and yet no study has shown estrogen to reverse this condition. We know that estrogen can help delay the onset of osteoporosis, but only temporarily. In 1999, the FDA finally eliminated osteoporosis as an indication for using estrogen.

They also claimed that estrogen is good for the heart. However, every long-term study of estrogen has indicated that it causes an increase in the incidence of heart attacks and strokes. It is contra-indicated in coronary artery disease and cerebrovascular disease, so I fail to see the claimed benefit of estrogen in these conditions.

In order to determine once and for all the benefits of long-term treatment with estrogen, the largest study ever of hormone replacement therapy was conducted, beginning in 1997. Called the Women's Health Initiative, it involved tracking the health of about 162,000 women. It was proposed as an eight-year study to monitor women on Premarin/Provera therapy. There was a side study of Premarin by itself among women who did not have a uterus.

Two years into the study they started getting some alarming statistics, but they continued with the research. However, after 5 ½ years it was decided to stop the study for ethical reasons. The data was showing a significantly higher number of aggressive-type breast cancers along with a higher incidence of cardiovascular complications in those women on the Premarin/Provera combination.

When the Premarin/Provera arm of the study was halted in the summer of 2002, it was front page news in every paper in America; it was the cover story of all the news magazines and became fodder for TV news programs and talk shows. For the first time in history, women were made aware of a truth that had been known in some circles for 30 years: that estrogen replacement therapy might not be safe.

The consistent recommendation put forth in the media was: go talk to your health care practitioner. However, if doctors had been aware of the similar results found by prior studies done in the 1990s, they might not have started their patients on these drugs in the first place or continued them.

Their responses to their patients' concerns about the study's findings ran along the lines of: "Don't worry about it" or "The benefits outweigh the risk" (they don't) or "It's your decision."

The other arm of the study, Premarin by itself, was stopped in March of 2004 because, once again, the risks proved to outweigh the potential benefits.

SUZANNE SOMERS — THE PROS AND CONS

Into this morass of contradictory information about hormones walked celebrity/author Suzanne Somers. With her book *The Sexy Years,* published in 2004, and a follow-up book called *Ageless,* published in 2006, Ms. Somers propelled herself into position as the new advocate for hormone replacement therapy.

Her books demonstrated some amazingly positive attributes. For the first time in history, women at large were made aware of bio-identical hormones—natural hormones that are identical to their own hormones and can be obtained from compounding pharmacies. No longer did they have to subject themselves to synthetic drugs that mimic hormones, nor did they have to take hormones appropriate for horses rather than humans.

Another tremendous benefit of Ms. Somers' books was their insistence that women have to become pro-active about their health; they cannot rely on the traditional medical system to keep them healthy.

However, Ms. Somers makes some points in her books that I feel require clarification.

First off, just because a hormone is bio-identical does not necessarily mean that it is safe. Hormones are extremely potent substances and must be used judiciously. Some of the doctors who Ms. Somers interviewed are very strong proponents of estrogen. She quotes one doctor as stating that the only time a woman is healthy is when she is having her periods. To achieve this aim, this doctor provides her post-menopausal patients with exceptionally high levels of estrogen in order to have them re-start menstruation. She has patients in their 80s and 90s bleeding every month and bent over with menstrual cramps. These women, needless to say, are intentionally put into the dangerous condition of estrogen dominance.

> *Women never stop making estrogen.*
> *Women do stop making progesterone.*

In my own practice, the sickest women I have ever seen are those who had been estrogen dominant, or were estrogen dominant when I first met them.

Let me remind you that anytime you utilize either a hormone or a drug, you have to weigh the benefits versus the risks. I look at estrogen as primarily a toxic hormone. It is known to cause six different cancers in women: breast, uterine, ovarian, cervical, vaginal, and colon cancers. It may cause Alzheimer's disease, strokes, heart attacks, and phlebitis with fatal pulmonary emboli. It may cause fibroids, endometriosis, adhesions, fibrocystic disease, asthma, migraine headaches, and gallbladder disease. It can lead to auto-immune diseases, such as lupus, rheumatoid arthritis, Hashimoto's thyroiditis, and others.

Estrogen is the hormone that causes women to experience menstrual cramps, PMS, breast tenderness, and nausea when they are pregnant. To add insult to injury, estrogen is lipogenic. It creates fat around the hips, thighs, and buttocks, and it is the cause of cellulite. Try telling women with a number of these problems that they are healthy because they are having periods and you might find yourself in an argument.

It is surprising to me that Suzanne Somers, who already had estrogen-induced breast cancer (she used to call estrogen her "happy pills"), is proposing that women take what I consider exceedingly high levels of estrogen. Not a week goes by when I do not see a patient who had an estrogen-induced cancer while they were still having their periods. In other words, their own estrogen caused these cancers—it does not get more "bio-identical" than your own hormones.

Interestingly, every problem, every complication, every downside to estrogen is eliminated by progesterone (not to be confused with Provera, or medroxyprogesterone, a synthetic chemical having no relationship to natural progesterone). Any time high levels of estrogen, such as those proposed by Suzanne Somers' books, are prescribed, a sufficient amount of progesterone must be prescribed to be protective. I believe the levels of progesterone recommended in her books are woefully inadequate and inappropriately administered.

My advice on the proper dosing is available in chapter 11. Two basic principles on which I base my approach are:

1. Women never stop making estrogen—it is probably the only hormone that hardly ever has to be replaced. It continues to be made by fat cells, skin cells, and the adrenal glands.

2. Women do stop making progesterone. Because of this, they are always at risk for developing breast cancer, uterine cancer, ovarian cancer, colon cancer, and other cancers from estrogen.

MY APPROACH

When certain hormone levels decrease, for either natural or surgical reasons, the pituitary responds by putting out certain hormones of its own to stimulate the ovaries to make more hormones. (The pituitary and hypothalamus glands are the structures of the brain that control other glands throughout the body.) In this case, the pituitary puts out a hormone called luteinizing hormone (LH) to stimulate the ovaries to make more hormones. LH may be the primary cause of the vascular symptoms women experience when they are going through menopause—the hot flashes and night sweats.

It is my feeling that the pituitary's primary reason for trying to raise ovarian hormone levels is so the woman can get pregnant. Once the pituitary is convinced a woman no longer needs to procreate, it stops sending out the signals and the hot flashes and related symptoms disappear. However, if the woman is placed on high levels of replacement hormones, the pituitary gets confused. It becomes convinced again that the woman is trying to get pregnant, and so whenever there is a significant drop (e.g., from stopping Premarin), it puts out LH and the symptoms recur.

The ovaries put out four different hormones—estrogen, progesterone, testosterone, and DHEA. Replacement of any or all of these hormones can alleviate perimenopausal and menopausal symptoms. The primary aim of the replacement of hormones is to keep the woman healthy and to prevent the body from deteriorating.

Since I look at estrogen as a potentially toxic and fat-creating hormone, and since the body never stops making estrogen, I take a relatively sparing approach to its use. I primarily prescribe estrogen for several reasons—to help alleviate hot flashes or night sweats, to help with "brain fog," and to relieve vaginal dryness. I will be discussing dosages, along with the various types of natural bio-identical estrogen available, in chapter 11. About two years prior to menopause women stop ovulating, which means they stop producing progesterone. This causes them to experience an increase in PMS, breast tenderness, cramps, and related symptoms. There may be a development of fibroids or fibrocystic disease in the breast, both being conditions caused by estrogen when there is not enough progesterone.

Progesterone is one of the most important hormones in a woman's body and, in my view, is probably the only hormone that has to be replaced after menopause. Testosterone and DHEA are two other hormones I often prescribe for my patients. I discuss the usual recommended dosages and applications in chapter 11.

THE BENEFITS OF PROGESTERONE

Looking over the stories of my patients presented in this book, you can see that even though they had various medical problems, every one of them had conditions related to a deficiency of progesterone. Keep in mind that every problem related to estrogen is created by a progesterone deficiency. Giving women natural progesterone takes away menstrual cramps, PMS, breast tenderness, menstrual migraines, and asthma. It prevents fibroids, endometriosis, fibrocystic disease, and estrogen-induced cancers.

The benefits of progesterone after menopause are as follows: It can eliminate hot flashes and prevent and treat osteoporosis. It is a natural anti-depressant—it is the feel-good hormone for women. Progesterone is thermogenic—it helps fat to burn. It prevents Alzheimer's disease, is great for the heart, and restores the libido (estrogen does nothing for the libido).

Throughout this book are numerous references to the benefits of progesterone in terms of preventing estrogen-induced cancer. It helps eliminate attention deficit disorder (ADD) and is the number one hormone for lowering insulin levels, thereby helping to prevent obesity and adult-onset diabetes.

WHAT ABOUT TESTOSTERONE?

The ovaries are the primary (but not the only) source of testosterone in women. My feeling is that testosterone is the second most important hormone to be replaced, after progesterone. Again, it certainly is a lot more important to replace than estrogen. In women, testosterone is the main hormone that prevents Alzheimer's (progesterone is second). It is the number one hormone for preventing and treating osteoporosis (progesterone is second). It is the number one hormone for the heart because there are more testosterone receptor sites in heart muscle than in any other tissue (250,000 people die of congestive heart failure every year, caused by weakening of the heart muscle). You cannot build muscle without testosterone, so it helps keep muscles toned; it gives women more energy and makes them feel more assertive. Testosterone is also necessary for an interest in sex; women often begin fantasizing about sex around 6 weeks after starting on testosterone and progesterone.

Another benefit of testosterone is that it can, when used correctly, that is, when used in tandem with certain exercises, eliminate urinary incontinence in about six days.

DHEA—THE ANTI-AGING HORMONE

Forty percent of the DHEA in a woman's body is produced by the ovaries; the other 60 percent comes mainly from the adrenals. However, as time passes, a woman's DHEA levels go down.

This hormone is an important part of the immune system and helps to prevent cancer, heart disease, and arthritis. Women with the highest levels of DHEA have the lowest incidence of breast cancer. DHEA also helps to prevent the "bad" cholesterol (LDL) from oxidizing. It is a precursor to estrogen and testosterone, so it can help to alleviate hot flashes. It is also considered a fat-burning hormone.

Surprisingly, even though DHEA is a very powerful hormone, it can be purchased over the counter as a food supplement in drug and health food stores. This by itself is a testament to the lack of information about hormones among medical practitioners. Like any other hormone, it should be used correctly, and only if there is a deficiency.

HORMONES FOR WOMEN—
THE "HOW-TO" CHAPTER

CHAPTER ELEVEN

The replacement of natural hormones is not an exact science. It requires a team approach among the patient, the doctor, and the compounding pharmacist.

Over time, dosages may have to be adjusted, based not so much on lab tests as on symptoms. For one thing, hormone levels can vary through the course of the day. For another, every person's hormone pattern is unique; there is no one-size-fits-all dosage. However, there are certain truisms. For instance, it's fair to generalize that in postmenopausal women, the estrogen level is lower but estrogen is still being produced, testosterone levels are much lower, DHEA levels are at least 40 to 50 percent lower, and progesterone levels are virtually non-existent.

The dosages and protocols that I recommend in this book are based on feedback from and experience with the thousands of men and women I have treated. If you feel that a certain approach might be appropriate for yourself, make notes and discuss it with your doctor. If he or she feels comfortable with the suggestions, a prescription may be obtained, to be filled by a compounding pharmacy. These are regular pharmacies that also have pharmacists specially trained in compounding various pharmaceuticals, including natural bio-identical hormones.

If your doctor is reluctant to deal with natural hormones, I suggest contacting a compounding pharmacy and asking them to recommend a physician who is amenable to natural bio-identical hormone replacement therapy.

PROGESTERONE

Progesterone is the number one hormone that has to be replaced in most women as they approach and go through menopause. Doctors frequently say that if a woman doesn't have a uterus, she doesn't need progesterone. This is not correct. As we have seen, progesterone is an essential hormone for protection against cancer and for addressing a wide spectrum of medical conditions. The level of progesterone drops as a person ages. Replacing it as part of an HRT regimen can be a keystone to good health. The benefits of natural bio-identical progesterone have been stated repeatedly throughout this book. It is applied as a transdermal cream that is absorbed through the skin fairly rapidly. Giving hormones as a cream allows them to bypass the liver initially.

The problem with the oral form of bio-identical progesterone, as recommended in Suzanne Somers' books, *The Sexy Years* and *Ageless,* is that it goes directly to the liver and gets converted to another hormone called pregnanediol. The same thing happens with the oral progesterone called Prometrium. This too is bio-identical, but it converts to a different hormone.

Progesterone cream has to be applied to areas where the skin is thin so it is absorbed into the bloodstream, not into fatty tissue. The best place is the inside (not the outside) of the wrist area and lower forearm. Another site could be the upper chest (but not the breast). It should never be applied to the abdomen or thighs.

The prescription should read: "Progesterone 100 mg/¼ tsp. Apply ¼ tsp BID [twice a day]." I recommend using it twice a day, every day, morning and evening.

Some women experience tenderness of the nipples when they first start progesterone, since there are many progesterone receptor sites around the nipples. If this occurs, lower the dosage to ⅛ tsp, and later increase to a ¼ tsp dose as the tenderness diminishes.

Some women experience menstrual bleeding after starting progesterone. Progesterone does not cause bleeding, but it does "heal" the uterus, that is, it prepares the uterus for menstrual periods or for pregnancy. The only hormone that causes menstrual bleeding is estrogen, and if estrogen levels are high enough when a woman starts progesterone, bleeding may occur. But this too will pass after one or two months.

THE TREATMENT OF ESTROGEN DOMINANCE

Prior to menopause, all symptoms related to an over-production of estrogen, which include menstrual cramps, breast tenderness, PMS, migraine headaches, mood swings, and asthma, can be eliminated using natural progesterone. The dosage in this case is the same as for menopause: 100 mg/¼ tsp twice a day. For those patients who feel more comfortable mimicking how the body naturally produces hormones, they can skip the progesterone cream the first seven to ten days after their cycle starts. In fact, this is necessary for those women wishing to get pregnant.

FERTILITY

One of the areas, I believe, where modern medicine's tragic lack of hormonal knowledge is demonstrated is in the field of fertility. Please note the following:

1. The number one reason why women fail to get pregnant or have trouble getting pregnant is a low progesterone level.

2. The number one reason why women have miscarriages is a low progesterone level.

3. The only reason women experience nausea when they are pregnant is a low progesterone level (the nausea is actually caused by estrogen).

4. A frequent cause of premature birth is a low progesterone level.

5. The only cause of postpartum depression, also known as the "baby blues," is a drop in progesterone levels.

For women who want to be pro-active about their problems with fertility, conception. and maintaining their pregnancies, natural progesterone is often the answer. For those who wish to avoid the expense and pain of in vitro fertilization, why not try natural progesterone?

The uterus requires progesterone for the fertilized egg to implant. It requires progesterone to sustain the pregnancy. Cramps, PMS, and breast tenderness with the monthly cycle— all are classic symptoms indicative of low progesterone levels. Taking natural progesterone not only eliminates these symptoms but it "heals" the uterus, which allows pregnancy to occur.

In cases where conception is desired, I recommend the same dosage of progesterone: 100 mg/¼ tsp twice a day, applied topically to the inner forearm or wrist. Using this daily for two months gives the uterus a chance to fully "heal" and be well prepared for a pregnancy. At the onset of the third cycle, the progesterone can be stopped for ten days and then restarted. If the woman becomes pregnant, she should increase the amount of progesterone (to support the pregnancy) as soon as she knows conception has occurred. This is best done with a vaginal progesterone suppository, in a dose of 400 mg twice a day, which must be maintained for at least four months. It should be used frequently enough to prevent nausea. Around the fourth or fifth month, the placenta starts pouring out proges-terone, so the woman can discontinue the cream, but it may be wise to continue it through the whole pregnancy.

Every person's hormone pattern is unique; there is no one-size-fits-all dosage.

In my view, using high dosages of progesterone after becoming pregnant offers three exceptional benefits: 1) no feelings of nausea, 2) prevention of miscarriage, and 3) a highly intelligent, usually very happy baby. Progesterone is particularly important for brain function development. In this regard, it is my feeling that premature infants might also benefit from progesterone, since they are prematurely deprived of the normally high levels of progesterone put out by the placenta in the final weeks of pregnancy.

PERI/POSTMENOPAUSAL REPLACEMENT OF ESTROGEN

My approach to hormone replacement for women is admittedly different from most others. My mother died of breast cancer and had been on estrogen therapy, so I have reason to doubt the rationale for estrogen replacement. However, my recommendations are based soundly on medical logic, somewhat on intuition, and a lot on personal experience with thousands of patients. In the remainder of the chapter I discuss various aspects of hormone replacement for women and explain my approach to each one.

EARLY TESTING FOR HORMONE LEVELS

Testing hormone levels and starting a woman on bio-identical hormones while she is in perimenopause helps ease her transition into menopause, a time when her body's chemistry is shifting. If a woman is still having periods, the ideal time to do a panel is about seven days prior to the onset of her cycle. If her menopausal symptoms are mild, I will have her start using a progesterone cream, possibly testosterone cream, and possibly DHEA. My preferred approach is to try to eliminate symptoms like hot flashes or night sweats without using estrogen. (As we saw earlier, a reduction in estrogen as well as other hormones triggers the pituitary to release luteinizing hormone, which seems to be the cause of hot flashes.)

If symptoms are severe, however, I will add BiEst cream (a combination of 20% estradiol and 80% estriol) at a dosage of 1.25 mg/¼ tsp. This can be applied to the skin once or twice a day. As soon as the symptoms abate, I recommend gradually decreasing the dosage. The eventual aim is to stop the hormone if possible. Remember, that in my approach the woman is also using progesterone cream, which protects her against the negative effects of estradiol.

Women never stop making estrogen. It continues to be manufactured by their fat cells, skin cells, and the adrenal glands even after menopause. The majority of women I have treated have not required it. However, there are women who feel better with the replacement of estrogen.

For women who do not have a major problem with hot flashes but do have vaginal dryness, I also prescribe estriol cream, 2.5 mg/¼ tsp, along with a vaginal applicator. This is applied intra-vaginally on a daily basis until the dryness is gone, then it is used perhaps once a week or once every other week, depending on dryness.

FOR WOMEN ON ESTROGEN

As far as I can decipher, the primary clinical necessity for replacing estrogen is to achieve levels of estrogen high enough for a woman to get pregnant. Such high estrogen levels offer no other benefits to the human body that I am aware of.

When a woman takes high levels of replacement estrogen, especially for a number of years, the pituitary is tricked into thinking she is still trying to get pregnant. Stopping estrogen at this point often results in severe hot flashes and night sweats. Very often, coming off Premarin is like detoxing from heroin. In these cases my approach is to maintain estrogen usage but change to a natural bio-identical estrogen in the form of BiEst cream 1.25 mg/¼ tsp, used twice a day to start, then gradually trying to wean off of it.

The BiEst cream, of course, is taken in conjunction with the natural bio-identical formulations of other hormones that might be needed, such as progesterone, DHEA, and testosterone.

Let me repeat: Women never stop making estrogen—though admittedly, they do not continue making high enough levels to become pregnant. If getting pregnant is a woman's goal even though she is menopausal, then she should follow the advice of Suzanne Somers' physician and take high levels of estrogen. Of course, since there are no eggs left, getting pregnant might be tough.

It has been my observation that women who are thin are more likely to benefit from or require estrogen replacement, because they have fewer fat cells to produce it. Women who are over-weight are generally loath to take it because, in most cases, giving them any type of estrogen, whether synthetic or bio-identical, creates fat and prevents them from losing weight.

THE SECOND
MOST IMPORTANT HORMONE

As we have seen, progesterone, in my view, is the most important hormone in a hormone replacement regimen during and after menopause. Testosterone is the second most important hormone. As with estrogen, women continue to make testosterone as they age, but at reduced levels. The level of free testosterone (the biologically active form of testosterone) in a menopausal woman is usually around 1.6. pg/nl This compares to a level of 6.4 pg/nl during the teenage years.

The benefits of testosterone are manifold. This is the number one hormone needed by the bones for the prevention and treatment of osteoporosis. It is also the number one hormone for heart health. As I mentioned earlier, there are more testosterone receptor sites in heart muscle than anywhere else in the body. Some 250,000 deaths are attributed to congestive heart failure (weakening of the heart muscle) every year.

How many might be avoided with testosterone?

In addition, testosterone is probably the most important hormone for prevention of Alzheimer's disease. Also, you cannot build muscle without the use of testosterone. The more muscle one has, the better one is able to prevent fat from forming and skin from sagging.

A woman requires two hormones for a good libido—progesterone and testosterone. If her libido has been low, it may take about six weeks after starting these hormones for her interest in sex to kick in.

TESTOSTERONE AND URINARY INCONTINENCE

Urinary incontinence is a very common problem in many women. Any time they cough, sneeze, laugh, or run on the tennis court, urine dribbles out. This forces many women to resort to mini-pads. Discussions with their doctors lead to prescriptions for Detrol or Ditropan, drugs that focus on bladder function. Sometimes they are referred to urologists for bladder surgery. Quite often, perhaps more often than not, the medication and the surgery do not help. The reason is that the incontinence they are experiencing is often not a bladder problem. As women get older, the muscles around the urethra weaken and they cannot keep urine from leaking out of the bladder.

Natural testosterone cream is almost 100 percent effective for this problem. A bio-identical testosterone cream can be obtained from a compounding pharmacy, along with a vaginal applicator, and is inserted vaginally once a day in the morning. Two exercises must be done along with using the cream to insure effectiveness. The first exercise is stopping and starting the urine stream while urinating, which helps you target the exact muscles you are trying to build up. The contraction of these muscles is called the Kegel maneuver. The second is actually the same exercise but done in other contexts. The same muscles need to be compressed for about ten seconds, 20 to 30 times per day, primarily in the morning. This can be done while you're driving, sitting, watching television, or engaged in other activities.

In about six to seven days, most women will experience a complete resolution of the incontinence—if, besides using the cream, they do both sets of exercises. Once the incontinence is gone, the testosterone cream can be applied to the inner forearm.

The dosages I usually prescribe are: First month: 2% cream or gel, ⅛ tsp applied intra-vaginally (if necessary for incontinence) or ⅛ tsp to the forearm, daily. Second month and thereafter: 1% cream or gel, ⅛ tsp applied to the forearm on a daily basis.

The best way to gauge testosterone levels is by the libido. If you are experiencing a healthy libido, cut the dosage to two or three times per week. Too much testosterone can create side effects, such as acne, body hair growth, scalp hair loss, elevated cholesterol, or aggressive behavior.

DHEA — THE ANTI-AGING HORMONE

Forty percent of the DHEA produced in a woman's body is made by the ovaries. After menopause, the ovaries quit manufacturing this hormone. DHEA is considered the mother of all steroid hormones, since it is the precursor to other hormones, most notably estrogen and testosterone. Clearly, replacing this hormone alone can help to reduce hot flashes and night sweats and restore libido.

The primary source of the remaining 60 percent of DHEA is the adrenal glands, though DHEA production by the adrenals also declines over the years. People who have been exposed to high levels of stress during their life very often have low levels of DHEA.

As discussed earlier, DHEA is also known as an anti-aging hormone. There appears to be a direct correlation between levels of DHEA and longevity. People with the highest DHEA levels seem to live longer lives. Perhaps this is related to the fact that DHEA stimulates the production of human growth hormone (HGH), sometimes referred to as the "fountain of youth" hormone.

DHEA influences the immune system and helps prevent cancer and arthritis. It's also beneficial for the cardiovascular system. It has the same effect as the "good" cholesterol (HDL) on the "bad" cholesterol (LDL), in that it prevents its oxidation, which can cause damage to the coronary arteries.

It is also known as a fat-burning hormone. The most likely reason why it promotes weight loss is because it lowers insulin levels, just as progesterone and testosterone do.

DHEA tends to enhance one's feeling of well-being. However, as with any hormone, replacement should be correlated carefully with need. Because DHEA can convert into other hormones, it is absolutely necessary to check blood levels of this hormone prior to starting its use and to monitor them during usage. When measuring DHEA, it is best to test DHEA-S levels rather than DHEA levels.

Since DHEA levels change with age, so-called normal levels are fairly low after menopause. My preference is to replace DHEA to achieve levels consistent with those of women about 40 years of age, which is in the neighborhood of 250 mcg/dl. I start women whose levels are very low, around 30 or less, with a dosage of 25 mg a day. Women with levels around 100 I start at 12.5 mg a day. I recommend obtaining DHEA by prescription from a compounding pharmacy; then you are assured of receiving a pharmaceutical dosage in a sustained-release form. Buying DHEA over the counter is less reliable, since standards for regulating dosages are low or non-existent. Hormones are potent chemicals, and one should be careful when using them.

The most common side effect of DHEA is acne—an indication that most of the DHEA is being converted into testosterone. The remedy here, of course, is to cut back on the dosage or the frequency of administration. Another approach might be to switch to 7-keto DHEA, a form of DHEA that does not convert into testosterone. It may be available at a health food store or possibly at a compounding pharmacy. A suggested dosage is 100 mg/day. DHEA in any form is best taken at bedtime.

ANDROPAUSE—THE MALE MENOPAUSE

CHAPTER TWELVE

Although this fact is often over looked, men and women produce exactly the same hormones. And most hormone levels in men, just as in women, become lower as men get older. Since hormones affect every system of the body, profound changes occur as one ages. This shift in men, which begins around age 50, is known as andropause. Its characteristics include a drop in energy, libido, stamina, and joi de vivre, associated with weight gain around the middle.

Moreover, it is just as important for men to receive bio-identical hormone replacement as it is for women. The consequences of altered hormone levels in men may lead to conditions such as coronary artery disease, Alzheimer's disease, prostate cancer, osteoporosis, and depression.

TESTOSTERONE

Unquestionably, the most important hormone to be considered for replacement in men is testosterone. It is most often thought of as a sex hormone, and it is, but it has other functions that are probably more vital.

Testosterone is the main hormone for the prevention of Alzheimer's disease. Studies done by the National Institutes of Health have confirmed this.

It is the number one hormone affecting heart tissue, including the coronary arteries, the conduction system, and, most important, the heart muscle itself. There are more testosterone receptor sites in heart muscle than in any other muscle in the body. Two studies came out in 2003 demonstrating the use of testosterone in men who had massive heart attacks, a situation that almost always results in congestive heart failure (CHF), a weakening of the heart muscle resulting in the backup of fluid into the lungs and possibly the rest of the body. The men who received testosterone failed to develop CHF; those who did not went into heart failure.

The development of osteoporosis, although not as common in men as women, actually has more dire consequences in men. A fractured hip in a male, most commonly related to osteoporosis, is associated with a 25 percent mortality rate in the first year of occurrence. Testosterone prevents and reverses osteoporosis.

An extremely common consequence of low testosterone levels in men is the onset of depression. They lose their interest in life, and their energy levels go down. Replacement of testosterone brings back energy, restores lost strength and interest in life, and leads to the buildup of muscle.

Very often the libido returns too. I've seen male patients in their 70s who hadn't had sex in 25 years who, with testosterone replacement, began having sex on a daily basis. Of course, their partners' hormones had to be dealt with as well.

THE CORRECT USE OF TESTOSTERONE

As with any other hormone, testosterone must be used correctly, especially since testosterone can convert into other hormones that may cause other problems.

It is often beneficial to determine the blood levels of testosterone. The test for free testosterone level is the most important test in this regard, not the more frequently used test for total testosterone level. The free testosterone level indicates the amount of biologically active testosterone that is available. However, levels of testosterone go up and down during the day.

The highest levels occur early in the morning, before testing is usually done. I have found that most men after the age of 50 have a level either below the normal range or else in the lower range of normal. Yet many of these men still get morning erections (an excellent indication of adequate testosterone levels) and have no problems with performance or libido.

No matter how low the level, if a man has no sexual problems I do not replace testosterone. Normal levels of free testosterone range from 50 to 210. Normal levels of total testosterone range from 250 to 1,000. I find that checking levels of testosterone is more useful in determining correct replacement dosages—too much or too little.

When replacing testosterone, one should be aware that this hormone can be converted into other hormones that may have unpleasant consequences. One is the form of estrogen known as estradiol, which can cause prostate cancer and possibly colon cancer. The other is dihydrotestosterone (DHT), which may cause prostate enlargement and male pattern hair loss.

Because of these possibilities, the levels of these two hormones should be monitored. High levels of DHT can often be avoided by correct placement of testosterone cream or gel on the skin. It is always best to apply testosterone to areas of the body devoid of hair. Certain enzymes found around hair follicles can convert testosterone into DHT (in other words, applying the cream to a shaved area will not help). Acceptable areas may include the upper and inner arms, shoulders, back of the knees, and around the ankles. Certain supplements can also help in this regard, among them saw palmetto, beta-sitosterol, and pygeum.

There are ways to keep estradiol levels lower. Discuss with the compounding pharmacist or your medical doctor the addition of 10 percent chrysin to the testosterone cream. Chrysin is an aromatase inhibitor. Aromatase is necessary to convert testosterone into estradiol, so anything that lowers this enzyme is beneficial. Arimidex can be used to lower estradiol. The recommended dose for men is 50 mcg per day, available from a compounding pharmacy.

Zinc is another important supplement to use while on testosterone. The prostate gland absorbs more zinc than any other area of the body. Zinc also acts as an aromatase inhibitor, thereby keeping estrogen levels low. As a side note: the eyes are second in the absorption of zinc, which helps prevent macular degeneration, the most common cause of adult blindness.

The dosage of testosterone should usually be about ¼ tsp of a 10 percent transdermal cream twice a day. The prescription should read: "Testosterone 10%. Apply ¼ tsp BID [twice a day] to hairless area" (upper or inner arms, shoulders, back of knees, or ankles). When the libido returns, one dose a day may be adequate.

Blood tests that should be monitored include:

- Total testosterone
- Free testosterone

- Estradiol
- DHT
- PSA (prostate specific antigen) with free PSA

The benefits of testosterone far outweigh any potential downside. But it should be used safely with attention to prostate health. In addition, too much testosterone can raise cholesterol levels, cause male pattern baldness, raise levels of red blood cells, and possibly cause aggressive behavior.

WHY PROGESTERONE

Many people, even some physicians, do not consider progesterone to be a male hormone (it is), and some are not aware that men produce estrogen (they do). Once again, men and women produce exactly the same hormones, but in different amounts. I prescribe progesterone for most of my male patients over 50 for a number of reasons. As men get older, their levels of progesterone decrease, becoming almost nonexistent around the age of 50. This is about the same age when men start putting on their "middle-aged paunch." Could there be a connection?

The answer is a most definite yes. And the reason? Progesterone is the number one hormone for lowering insulin levels, the hormone that creates fat right around the middle. This is also the time of life when men may experience fatigue between 3 and 4 in the afternoon or getting sleepy while driving or after eating—the classic times for tiredness related to over-production of insulin. When insulin levels go up, blood sugar goes down.

A brain deprived of sugar gets sleepy. The number one cause of people falling asleep while driving is hypoglycemia. The number one cause of hypoglycemia is too much insulin.

The number one cause of too much insulin is low progesterone. One of the first benefits people experience after starting progesterone is that they no longer get sleepy in the afternoon, after eating, or while driving.

Another reason I believe men over 50 should take progesterone is that I suspect that it prevents prostate cancer. I cannot point to studies that show this, but it is logical. As men approach andropause, their progesterone levels drop and their estrogen levels start rising. This is also about the time that prostate cancer becomes a risk. If estrogen causes six different cancers in women, why wouldn't it be up to no good in men as well? Not only cancer of the prostate but also cancer of the colon could be caused by excess estrogen in men's bodies.

Other benefits from progesterone in men are as follows: prevention of Alzheimer's disease, prevention of osteoporosis, prevention of coronary artery spasm, reversal of depression, and elimination of asthma.

JIM B.'S STORY

The dramatic effects of progesterone in men are perhaps best illustrated by the story of one of my patients, Jim B. When I first met Jim, he was 54 years old. He came into my office, sat down, and with no other preamble stated, "Doc, if you don't help me, I'm going to commit suicide." He added that I was his last resort.

He had four major complaints: 1) he was (obviously) depressed, 2) he was severely hypoglycemic, 3) he had asthma, and 4) he had osteoporosis.

I told him right off that his problems were easily resolved and that he had a deficiency of progesterone. He looked at me quizzically and said that over the previous several years he had been back and forth across the country, spent tens of thousands of dollars, consulted with the best doctors in the finest clinics and institutions, had hundreds of blood tests and procedures done, and no one had ever mentioned the word "progesterone," much less tested for it. And here, in the space of several minutes, I identified this as his problem.

Although he strongly suspected I was a "quack," he agreed to a trial of progesterone. In only three days he was saying, "In my entire life I have never felt so good."

This response was exactly the response I had expected. Progesterone affects every neurotransmitter in the brain and can readily eliminate depression. It prevents the over-production of insulin and helps hypoglycemia. It is wonderful for eliminating asthma. This may possibly be related to its anti-estrogen effect. Estrogen is a common cause of asthma, and men often have high levels of estrogen. Progesterone is also beneficial for preventing and treating osteoporosis.

During their training, doctors receive an extremely limited amount of information about hormones. Thus it is not surprising that every medical specialist Jim had spoken to was unable to diagnose his problem.

I consider progesterone the second most important hormone for replacement in men. There are actually no downsides to using this hormone. It must be obtained from a compounding pharmacy. The cream is used in lieu of an oral form in order to bypass the liver. The prescription I usually recommend is: progesterone 100 mg/¼ tsp twice a day for two weeks, then ¼ tsp once a day. Progesterone is best applied to the wrist area and lower forearm. However, men who greatly over-produce insulin may require dosages three times a day.

I have only had one complaint from a male patient whom I placed on progesterone. He said it made him too compassionate. Wives, are you listening?

In all fairness, I should mention that Jim B. had ADHD.

As I describe in chapter 15, the chapter on ADD and ADHD, these patients have high levels of adrenaline to combat their persistent hypoglycemia induced by high insulin levels. Adrenaline is the "anger hormone." Giving Jim progesterone lowered his insulin levels, so he no longer had hypoglycemia, and he stopped pouring out adrenaline (i.e., he became "compassionate").

Progesterone also eliminates restless leg syndrome (RLS), another condition caused by too much adrenaline, although this is not recognized by the medical community. Doctors claim there is no known cause for this condition and that it is incurable. They treat it with toxic anti-Parkinsonian drugs, once again treating the symptoms instead of the cause. However, using progesterone often eliminates RLS in about one week.

Adults with ADHD, RLS, fibromyalgia—all conditions associated with too much adrenaline—usually require progesterone three times a day and must cut back on their carbohydrate intake to reduce sugar and insulin levels.

WHAT ABOUT DHEA?

The primary concern related to DHEA is that it can raise the level of estradiol, the hormone associated with prostate cancer and possibly colon cancer. However, when DHEA is given in correct dosages this rarely happens. The intent of hormone replacement therapy is simply to replace what's missing, not to add more than is necessary. The number of receptor sites available for each hormone is limited, so extremely high doses can cause problems.

The correct lab test for assessing blood levels of DHEA is the test for DHEA-S (not plain DHEA). Most men in their 50s have levels around 175 or less. My goal in replacing

DHEA is to achieve the levels that were present around the age of 40. This means a DHEA-S level of around 400–500. For men with levels of less than 100, I give a dosage of 50 mg a day. For levels higher than 100, I start with a 25 mg dosage. DHEA is best taken in the evening.

THOUGHTS ABOUT PROSTATE CANCER

Allowed a long-enough life span, most men will develop prostate cancer. Statistically, however, only 7 percent of prostate cancers will metastasize. In essence, this means that if a prostate cancer is left alone, most men would die with it and not from it.

Based on this information, watchful waiting appears to be a feasible and logical approach when it comes to prostate cancer. This disease is diagnosed by sticking twelve to eighteen needles into the prostate, which means some blood capillaries will be pierced and disturbed. If there are cancer cells present, is it possible, then, that the biopsy procedure itself may cause the cancer to metastasize by allowing cancer cells to get into the blood?

The traditional thinking in medicine is that testosterone is the hormone that causes prostate cancer. Yet the men with the highest levels of testosterone have the lowest incidence of prostate cancer. And if it were true, why wouldn't males have prostate cancer at the age of 17, when the levels of testosterone are at their highest?

The level of testosterone in men starts dropping when they are in their 20s, becoming very low by the age of 50. While this is happening, the level of estradiol is rising. Men in their 50s and beyond almost always have higher levels of estrogen than women have. And they are no longer producing proges-terone to protect them from all of this estrogen.

Keep in mind that estrogen is the only known cause of uterine cancer (other than the drug Tamoxifen). Since the prostate is derived embryologically from the exact tissue that the uterus comes from, why wouldn't estrogen also be causing prostate cancer? Logically, it would appear to be so. Yet, in some cases, estrogen is used to treat prostate cancer.

> *In my view, prostate cancer is probably a disease to be prevented, rather than to be treated, by balancing a man's hormones and prescribing appropriate supplements.*

Right now, testosterone is thought to cause cancer of the prostate, so most of the attention in treating prostate cancer is on eliminating testosterone. Often the drug Lupron is administered, and many times it appears to be beneficial. However, besides lowering testosterone levels, it also eliminates estradiol. Perhaps this is its main benefit. Interestingly, in Europe testosterone is now being used to treat prostate cancer.

In my view, prostate cancer is probably a disease to be prevented, rather than to be treated, by balancing a man's hormones and prescribing appropriate supplements. Here is a list of some of the supplements known to prevent and/or treat prostate cancer:

- Vitamin D3 – 5,000 I.U./day for prevention, 20,000 I.U./day for treatment
- Vitamin E – 800 I.U./day in the form of mixed tocopherols
- Lycopene – 30 mg/day
- Selenium – 200 mcg/day
- Zinc – 25–50 mg/day

- Indole-3-carbinol – 300 mg/day
- Beta-sitosterol – 300 mg/day

Note that Vitamin D3 is known to prevent 26 different cancers; it also kills cancer cells. It is more likely a prohormone, a substance that converts into a hormone, rather than a vitamin. Dosages of up to 50,000 I.U./day are probably safe.

For men whose lab tests show an elevated PSA (prostate specific antigen) it is imperative to check the free PSA level as well. A PSA level greater than 2.5 is now considered elevated (not 4.0, as previously thought). The free PSA test is an important determinant of the possibility of cancer. However, keep in mind that the most common cause of an elevated PSA level is benign prostatic hypertrophy (BPH). Another frequent cause is prostatitis (infectious or inflammatory).

A free PSA percentage greater than 20 percent suggests the absence of cancer; a level less than 10 percent suggests its presence. Levels from 11 to 20 percent are in the gray area.

When my patients show any elevation of PSA, I start them on progesterone, prescribe the supplements just listed, and continue to track their PSA and free-PSA levels. This approach is my own. Please discuss any prostate concerns you have with your own physician.

ADULT-ONSET DIABETES AND LOUIS R.

CHAPTER THIRTEEN

Louis R. is a successful and contented 60-year-old who has struggled with weight all his life. When I took his family history, it became clear that his weight problem was genetic. Everyone in his family—mother, father, aunts, uncles, grandparents—was "heavyset."

When we talked about his goals, Louis emphasized that he was bound and determined not to "let himself go" at age 60, the way many of his family members had done.

When his treatment is completed, Louis can be assured he'll be able to control his weight without dieting. He'll also be able to manage his adult-onset diabetes without the use of medication. Here is his story:

I am a type II diabetic. My diabetes started in middle age, but even before that I'd always experienced problems with my weight. At six different times in my life I've been 40 pounds over-weight, and I've dieted to lose those 40 pounds. Each time I was successful in losing the weight, but over time those same 40 pounds reappeared. I have done Weight Watchers, I used Diet Center twice, and I've gone the Nutra System route and others. Each of these diets was effective. The pounds just flew off but psychologically I was about four feet off of the ground at all times. Either that or I was unbearably fatigued. My whole family is predisposed to being heavy. My father was a little shorter than me and at one time weighed about 240 pounds. My paternal grandmother was about six feet tall and a very big woman who weighed about 230 pounds. When my late sister was diagnosed with colon cancer, she weighed 290 pounds. My maternal grandfather was large, as was my maternal grandmother.

So I'm from sturdy big stock and I'm never going to be one of those men who weigh 165 pounds. I know that. Once I dieted my way down to 168 pounds but I looked horrible. People were asking me what disease I had, I was so gaunt. Today my goal is more realistic. I want to reach 185 pounds and stay there for the rest of my life. My other goal is to control my diabetes with diet and exercise.

When my mother turned 60, she told me she just wanted to be a fat old lady. She just let everything go. When she died she was 5'2" and weighed about 240 pounds. I turned 60 last year and I decided I do not want to be like my mother. I'm going in the opposite direction. I want to slim down and build some muscle and remain attractive.

I have to say up front that when I first visited Dr. Platt, I walked into his office with an attitude of skepticism. Not because of all the diets I'd gone on, but because I have an insider's knowledge of medical scams. For 20 years my career consisted of marketing and selling pharmaceutical products. I know what pharmaceutical companies will stoop to in order to turn a profit. I lost my innocence about medicine long ago, and I'm always on the lookout for someone trying to turn an easy buck.

But once I spoke to Dr. Platt I was relieved. From the way he talked, I realized he wasn't just promoting products. What he said about why people hang onto weight and why their bodies hate to lose fat made sense. There was none of the jargon and medical babble that tends to cluster around trendy medical scams.

Platt's office staff have also been very supportive, and they communicate a sense of being genuinely interested in everyone who comes in there. The whole atmosphere is wonderful. They're not punitive when you don't meet your goals as expected.

As far as the process of losing weight is concerned, it's been virtually painless. The diet itself is easy to follow. I'm a fruit freak and that's been the most difficult thing to give up, but I realize that I will be able to go back to fruit later in the process; it's not something I have to give up for the rest of my life. Once I've lost the weight I want to lose, the fruit will be re-introduced. In the short term, trust me, if that's all I have to give up, that's fine.

There was a brief period when I was losing weight but not feeling very energetic. I went in to see one of the nutritional counselors, who recommended a multi-mineral. It was my thought, knowing just enough about medicine to be dangerous, that perhaps I should be taking potassium. I know diets can be potassium-depleting. But the counselor said not only to do potassium but to take a multi-mineral as well. Sure enough, my energy returned and I started feeling absolutely great. It made me wonder whether I'd been lacking in some mineral or other for many years.

During my very first interview with Dr. Platt it came out that my sister died of colon cancer and that now one of her daughters has colon cancer. Also, my mother had a mastectomy when she was 38. Dr. Platt was very interested in this. It's one of the reasons why he placed me on progesterone, which is erroneously thought of as a female hormone. But according to him, progesterone will protect me from the excess estrogen I'm putting out. He knew that was true even before he did my blood work, just from my family medical history.

I was also started on testosterone, and the amounts were very carefully monitored by Dr. Platt's office. It certainly helped with *my libido (interest in sex). According to the blood work my DHEA is that of a 30-year-old. Dr. Platt wanted to know if anyone in my family had lived a long time. My grandfather lived to almost 90, and my mother was almost 90 when she died.*

Dr. Platt also thought my thyroid was not putting out as much hormone as it should, so he has me on a couple of thyroid medications. This makes a difference. I've noticed since I've been on this diet that I don't get that late afternoon letdown I used to get. I think that's due to the thyroid medications and the progesterone, which Dr. Platt states is stabilizing my blood sugar.

So far I've lost 32 pounds, and I've weaned myself off one of my medications for diabetes. As we go along we're fine-tuning my medications. It seems to be a rather sensible approach. I'm very pleased with the results.

DIABETES AND INSULIN

Louis has a strong family history of both obesity and adult-onset diabetes. This means everyone in his family over-produces insulin, and insulin is the hormone that creates fat.

A simple way of thinking about insulin is to understand that insulin will take any sugar the body's not using and store it primarily in the fat cells. Once the sugar is absorbed into the fat cells, it is converted into fat. People have a limited number of fat cells, which therefore can only contain a limited amount of fat. As these cells fill up with fat, it gets harder for insulin to get the sugar into them. This is what I refer to as "insulin resistance"; there are other types of insulin resistance that also play a significant role in diabetes. Whichever type is in effect, the body responds by producing even more insulin. This is called "hyperinsulinemia." Insulin not only creates fat, it prevents fat from getting out of the fat cells—it is a fat-storing hormone.

One can easily see that if you have too much insulin, you are going to have a weight problem.

Eventually the fat cells get completely filled up and sugar can no longer get into the fat cells—so it builds up in the bloodstream and the patient is told he or she has diabetes. While in fact diabetes is frequently a disease of too much insulin, doctors approach diabetes as if it is a disease of high blood sugar. So they give their patients medications to stimulate the pancreas to make even more insulin. This extra insulin literally pushes the sugar into the fat cells, creating even more weight gain.

The exception to this is the medication Glucophage, which goes by the generic name metformin. Glucophage doesn't actually lower blood sugar; it acts by increasing the sensitivity of tissues in the body to insulin, leading to a lowering of insulin levels. Needless to say, I do not necessarily wean people off this particular diabetic medication.

Many patients with type II (adult-onset) diabetes may inappropriately wind up on insulin injections. Since probably 90 percent of people with adult-onset diabetes already have too much insulin to begin with, placing them on insulin often exacerbates their weight problem.

HYPOGLYCEMIA AND INSULIN

If my patients are having hypoglycemic reactions, usually manifested as afternoon fatigue, sleepiness after eating, sleepiness while in a car either as the driver or as a passenger, this tells me that they are over-producing insulin, irrespective of blood sugar levels.

If I have a patient who has been diagnosed with diabetes and has symptoms suggesting hypoglycemia, I can assume they are producing an adequate amount of insulin. These patients can often be cured of their diabetes by lowering their insulin levels and changing the way they eat to a fat-burning meal plan. Once a certain amount of fat has been eliminated, there is room in the fat cells for the sugar to be taken in, and the diabetes condition is gone.

In my opinion, there is one major cause for hyperinsuline-mia (too much insulin), namely, too little progesterone. Louis' family history is classic for this condition—which underscores the importance of spending time talking to patients. Much information can be gleaned from a family history. In the first place, the prevalence of diabetes in the family was suggestive of Syndrome X, the form of hyperinsulinemia associated with high triglyceride levels and low HDL cholesterol. The strong family history of estrogen-related cancers also suggested low progesterone levels.

HORMONAL INFLUENCES

Louis had significant hormone problems. Besides indicating low progesterone levels, his family history was consistent with evidence of estrogen dominance. The history of colon cancer and breast cancer among the women in his family would have been related to estrogen. The low progesterone led to problems with hyperinsulinemia, with resultant obesity.

Blood tests indicated that Louis also had low levels of testosterone. This too is a hormone that lowers insulin levels, just like progesterone. Testosterone is probably the most important hormone to replace in a male, for multiple reasons. It treats and prevents osteoporosis (as we have seen, fractured hips are associated with a 25 percent mortality rate in men). It appears to help prevent Alzheimer's disease. And a man is not able to perform sexually with low levels of testosterone.

Testosterone also helps keep the heart healthy: The heart muscle has more testosterone receptor sites than any other muscle, which means the heart uses more testosterone than any other organ. Testosterone is now being used to treat congestive heart failure in men. A man cannot build muscle without testosterone. It has been found that many men (and women) have very low levels of testosterone after a heart attack. Could it be a contributing factor?

DIABETES AND WEIGHT MANAGEMENT

Louis will probably have to restrict the carbohydrates in his diet for the rest of his life. Making Louis aware of how his metabolism works—how sugar and insulin throw his energy levels out of whack, and how he can use protein to stabilize his system—has made all the difference. With his hormones balanced and with an informed approach to his diet, Louis is able to manage his weight and avoid the pitfalls of diabetes.

We have a nationwide epidemic of obesity and type II diabetes. Both of these conditions are strictly hormonal problems. Understanding this connection, one can appreciate once again the miraculous benefits of restoring hormonal balance with bio-identical hormones.

PSYCHOGENIC MEDICATION AND GREG C.

CHAPTER FOURTEEN

When Greg C. walked into my office, I saw a handsome 32-year-old whose body had become distorted by weight gain. He talked earnestly and honestly about a recent nervous breakdown and the four powerful psychogenic drugs—almost all of them lipogenic (causing the body to store fat)—doctors said he needed for mental balance. I want him to tell his story for the benefit of the millions of people taking anti-depressants and other psychogenic drugs who could live normal, happy lives if their hormones were balanced.

I've always been a high achiever. I set goals for myself and then I pursue them with everything I've got. For a long time this worked well for me. My achievements were pleasing to my parents, who gave me a lot of approval and made me want to achieve even more. My father was very successful financially at a young age and placed a lot of value on worldly status and possessions. So did my mother, and, of course, so did I.

By my mid-20s I was making a lot of money working in the hospitality business in Las Vegas. I had a responsible job at Caesar's Palace and I gave it everything I had, so much so that I was losing my balance. I worked so much that I stopped doing very much of anything else. Las Vegas is a 24-hour-a-day, 365-days-a-year place, a city that never sleeps, and demands are made on you constantly to keep the machinery running. I would always go the extra mile to troubleshoot an emergency, accommodate unexpected guests … whatever came up.

Somehow, amidst all this work I did manage to meet a woman I wanted to spend my life with. Stephanie and I married when I was 30 and she got pregnant soon afterwards. This added even more responsibility, and although I didn't understand it then I began showing signs of nervous exhaustion.

I began to lose my appetite. I'm a wonderful cook—I went to school to become a chef early in my life—and every day after work I'd come home and cook a healthy meal for my wife while she was pregnant, but I found I couldn't eat. After the baby was born—he's a boy—I cooked for each of them the kinds of nutritious meals I felt they should have, but again I couldn't eat the food I cooked. I'd have a piece of toast or something. For someone going at breakneck speed the way I was, this wasn't good. I wasn't taking care of myself.

You see, I had this Superman complex where I felt I had to take care of everyone and everything. I never told my wife how scared I was of failing because that wouldn't be taking care of her. I hid my insecurities and just pushed myself.

Often I'd go back to work after dinner. If my wife protested, I'd make up a story about some emergency that had come up. The truth was I felt I had to do more just to keep up. It's a mindset. I felt things would fall apart if I didn't hurry up and do more.

At a certain point this became an issue for me and Stephanie, and we saw a counselor who suggested I work in a less stressful environment. I found a job at the Las Vegas Convention and Visitors' Authority, thinking it would allow me more time for a normal life. But just the opposite happened. I became even more stressed and worked even longer hours. Even with my son at home I couldn't tear myself away from work.

Stephanie insisted I see a psychiatrist about my workaholic attitude. I began seeing a woman who diagnosed me as bi-polar and gave me three strong medications to even out my highs and lows. I began talk therapy as well.

Looking back, I probably should have gotten a second opinion from another psychiatrist. The talk therapy only dealt with my euphoria and my depression. We never talked about the underlying problems that were driving me. I began getting worse and worse. I felt so much responsibility that I couldn't handle it. There was nothing in my life that felt comfortable and grounded. I felt anxious all the time; I couldn't sleep or eat.

At one point I threatened to drive to Hoover Dam and jump. Stephanie got on her knees and cried and begged me to get some real help. There is a psychiatric hospital in Connecticut my family knows about and they offered to send me there. By now I'd lost my job. I knew that if I wanted to get my life on track I'd have to get more help.

So I spent the summer in Connecticut getting a lot of individual counseling, and group therapy, too. Stephanie went to Chicago with our son to stay with her parents. We lost our house. Stephanie is now in Chicago and we are both praying for reconciliation and a chance to start life over together.

In Connecticut they added lithium to the drugs I was taking, bringing the number to four. These were all very strong drugs, including Effexor, Paxil, and Depakote. I didn't like the way I felt on the drugs. They made me drowsy and blurred my thinking.

Another side effect was weight gain. I went from my habitual 165 pounds (I'm 6 feet tall) up to 215.

When I left the psychiatric hospital, I came to the desert to stay with my mother. Today I'm under the care of a psychiatrist, going through a healing process. When I told a friend about how uncomfortable I felt weighing 215, he recommended I see Dr. Platt.

Initially I went just for the weight loss, but I have received so much more from my treatment. The great miracle is that not only have I gone back to my usual weight, I've been able to wean myself off all the drugs I was on.

My intake interview with Dr. Platt made me feel very comfortable. When I told him about all the drugs 1 was taking, he told me I was over-medicated, and that if I followed his hormone treatment and his diet I would be able to wean myself off the drugs. I told my psychiatrist about Dr. Platt and he was open to the idea of helping the weaning process along, as long as I continued in therapy with him and continued to examine the issues that got me into trouble in the first place.

I started Dr. Platt's treatment in January and set myself the goal of being drug-free and at the proper weight by the end of March. I reached my goal by early March, and today feel absolutely fantastic. I feel so lucid and my thought processes are so clear compared to how I felt on the drugs.

I'm continuing in therapy and applying for jobs in various industries such as banking and insurance—more conventional industries where the hours are normal. I don't want to be in the hospitality business any more.

While I'm waiting for a job to come through, I'm delivering newspapers at night. It's something I never could have imagined myself doing at the age of 32. But it gives me time to think about what I want for my future, and I see the moon and stars every night and watch the sun rise every morning. It's a humbling experience, but it's also a rebirth. I feel the foundation of my house has been properly poured this time. I've gotten so much help with my worldview, both from my psychiatrist and from Dr. Platt, who encourages me to approach life as an enjoyable journey. I'm thinking in a way I've never thought before. I used to have so much fear that I was never going to amount to anything in life. Now I know that if I stay balanced I will have an impact on the lives of my loved ones and hopefully my community, and that's all I want.

THE DANGERS OF PSYCHOTROPIC MEDICATION

Greg's case is a classic example of how medications can contribute to a person's problems instead of helping them.

My approach with my patients is always to look for the underlying causes of their problems. I can't just look at the problems without seeing the entire person. Greg came to me for weight loss, but I did not want to treat him as a straightforward weight management patient without addressing those four incredibly powerful drugs he was taking. I knew that even if I were to get him down to his ideal weight, those drugs would eventually bring him right back to where he was. So it would make sense to address the psychogenic drugs first.

Although I'm not a psychiatrist, I found the diagnosis of bi-polar disorder suspicious. That's a very specific disorder— one that tends to be over-diagnosed, by the way. I didn't believe that Greg was really suffering from that malady. Since I know that hormones have a tremendous impact on the neurotransmitters in the brain, I decided to go on the working theory that Greg, like many people, was being diagnosed with something very serious when in fact he was probably just suffering from unbalanced hormones.

Whatever Greg's psychological difficulties were, I knew that with the right hormones he could get some relief from his symptoms. I told him that my goal was to get him off his drugs and to get his hormones in balance. He was delighted with that, since he felt foggy and uncomfortable on the medications.

Fortunately, Greg's psychiatrist was open to the idea of weaning him off of these powerful drugs. He felt that Greg's nervous breakdown was an extreme stress reaction, not a symptom of bi-polar disorder, and that if Greg could address his issues in talk therapy he could eventually go back to living a normal, drug-free life.

ADJUSTING GREG'S HORMONES

In my view, Greg's weight problem was caused by a combination of the medications he was on plus too much insulin. The fact that most of Greg's weight had settled in around his abdomen was a sign of over-producing insulin. So I started him on natural progesterone right away. I did this for four reasons:

- Progesterone reduces insulin
- Progesterone regulates blood sugar levels
- Progesterone is wonderful for brain tissue (progesterone levels are 20 times higher in brain tissue than anywhere else)
- Progesterone is a natural anti-depressant

Between progesterone and the meal plan, Greg began losing weight right away. With his psychiatrist's help, he slowly reduced the amount of Paxil, Effexor, Depakote, and lithium he was taking. As he continuously lowered the dosages of those lipogenic medications, his weight loss speeded up.

He got into a positive feedback loop whereby he liked the way he was looking, which led to feeling better about himself and making faster progress in talk therapy, which led to further success with his weight management program, and so on. As the weeks went by, you could see the transformation.

Eventually Greg returned to being the person he'd been before he started the medications, minus the driven, workaholic overlay. Today he's a very energetic, forward-looking man with a lot to live for.

Greg will eventually be reunited with his wife and child. With the help of hormones, he'll be able to live a balanced life that he truly enjoys. In addition, he is now acutely aware of the importance of balancing his son's hormones and his wife's hormones.

Greg's problems were strictly hormonal: too much adrenaline, too much insulin, too much cortisol, and too little progesterone. Putting them back into balance gave him the "miracle" he was looking for.

THE UNDERLYING PROBLEM

Greg's story illustrates why it is so important to understand the background of one's patients.

When I first talked with Greg, it was immediately apparent that he had a classic case of ADHD. Adults with this problem frequently become workaholics and type A personalities. These people are living on adrenaline. They start out with low progesterone levels, which causes an over-production of insulin. This leads to hypoglycemia and to an outpouring of adrenaline to bring sugar levels up.

This was Greg's underlying metabolic state. When he began working in Las Vegas, the new element of stress was added.

Now his adrenal glands were over-producing not only adrenaline but also cortisol (this is addressed in chapter 20). The cortisol raised his sugar levels, leading to even more insulin production. This led to more hypoglycemia, which led to more adrenaline. He lost his appetite because of the high levels of adrenaline, leading to a body starved for fuel, which created even more stress.

He did not have bi-polar disorder; he just had a major hormonal imbalance. One can readily see why sometimes psychological conditions can be treated with hormones in a more effective manner than with drugs.

ADD AND ADHD—
THE SILENT EPIDEMIC

CHAPTER FIFTEEN

I could not write a book about the influence of hormones without making special mention of attention deficit disorder (ADD) and attention deficit hyperactivity disorder (ADHD). In my view, these two conditions are primarily related to a hormonal imbalance involving high insulin and the resultant hypoglycemia, or low blood sugar.

There are many kids with symptoms of ADD who are struggling in school today because they have difficulties focusing. Often the reason they cannot pay attention in class or do homework is that they are hypoglycemic. Any time sugar is taken from the brain, the brain cannot focus. The reason for the low sugars is that the kids are over-producing insulin.

Because of the hypoglycemia these youngsters experience a persistent craving for foods that provide sugar, such as fruit juice, soda, and candy. And very often kids with ADD have a weight problem, since they are continuously eating high glycemic carbohydrates.

ADHD starts out the same way—too much insulin leading to low sugar levels. However, kids with ADHD have to contend with another hormone: adrenaline.

The brain cannot function without sugar, and the body has an amazing capacity for finding ways to raise the blood sugar level when it is low. Prominent among these regulatory reactions is a process called gluconeogenesis, which, simply put, creates sugar from protein. It is mediated through the sympathetic nervous system, which means the body pours out adrenaline to raise sugar levels. Adrenaline, which is natural speed, causes these kids to be hyperactive.

At the same time that the body is creating adrenaline, the low sugar levels are prompting cravings for food high in sugar. Ingestion of sugar then leads to the over-production of insulin, leading to a drop in sugar, leading to difficulty focusing, leading to the over-production of adrenaline, leading to hyper-active behavior, and on and on.

Kids with ADHD are usually thin. The hyperactivity burns up the sugar before it's converted to fat for storage. Oftentimes the hyperactivity is masked by the child's active involvement in sports.

Kids with ADHD are treated with drugs such as Ritalin, Adderal, and Strattera. However, approaching this condition from a hormonal standpoint in most cases eliminates ADHD without having to resort to medication.

You can probably guess that the missing hormone that can balance the high insulin and adrenaline levels and alleviate ADD and ADHD would be progesterone. We inherit our hormone levels from either parent. If a mother is estrogen dominant, she is also low in progesterone. This can be passed on to her daughter or son. Anyone with a low progesterone level will over-produce insulin, thereby causing hypoglycemia, leading to ADD.

AN AMAZING TRANSFORMATION

I should mention my experience with one nine-year-old child who had a classic case of ADHD. He had been thrown out of every public school in the city of Indio, California, for fighting with other children, shoving teachers, and similar behaviors. His mother was desperate because the boy sincerely wanted to go back to school. I do not treat young children with ADHD in my practice, but I made an exception in this case.

I talked with the boy and helped him understand that the sugar-based diet he had been eating and drinking was part of the problem. I told him he would be putting a cream on his lower forearm. He agreed to follow the protocol and was given a meal plan.

Twenty-four hours later, his mother told me she could not stop crying; she had never seen her son behave so well. He did ten pages of homework—quite an accomplishment for someone who had never done homework before. His ADHD was gone.

In spite of his recovery, the Indio school board refused to re-admit him into the system. I had written a two-page letter explaining that he was better, but the educational system, not surprisingly, proved to be blind to how simply ADHD can be addressed.

On the positive side, he is now attending a parochial school. His sixth-month report card was all A's—not surprising since most ADHD children are extremely intelligent.

When the boy went for his next therapy appointment, the psychiatrist, who had been following him for his ADHD, saw right away that the signs of the disorder were gone. But when he asked the mother what her son was taking and she told him natural progesterone cream, he told her to stop the cream immediately, that it was a female hormone, and to put her son back on the drugs that had been prescribed. She explained that the boy wouldn't take them because they made him feel sick. He told her to do it anyway. Needless to say, the mother continued with the cream.

I subsequently spoke with the psychiatrist, who refused to accept anything I was saying because there were no drug-company studies to verify it. He refused to allow his own powers of observation to see that progesterone was beneficial. Psychiatry developed purely as an observational science; now it is almost purely about psychopharmacology. He would rather place this nine-year-old boy on potentially lethal drugs, with multiple side effects, than use a natural bio-identical hormone with no side effects. His statement that progesterone is a female hormone is typical of the lack of education doctors receive about hormones.

As stated previously, I do not treat young children that are hyperactive in my practice—but I do treat their parents. If a parent has ADHD, there is a 50 percent chance that the child will also be hyperactive. If the child is adopted, then he or she has an even greater likelihood of having ADHD. This is because the majority of women who give up their children for adoption seem to be young mothers who have gotten into drugs and alcohol and gotten pregnant, and, in my opinion, most young people who get involved with drugs and alcohol have ADHD.

ADHD IN ADULTS

There are many adults with undiagnosed ADD or ADHD. People who experience sleepiness between 3 and 4 in the after-noon or while driving—this is ADD. I use the word "ADD" interchangeably with "hypoglycemia," because when the level of sugar in the brain is low, the person can't focus. People who become workaholics may actually have ADHD and are living on high levels of adrenaline caused by recurrent hypoglycemia.

Simply put, I view ADD and ADHD as a matter of too little progesterone, too much insulin, and, in the case of ADHD, too much adrenaline.

If you ask a specialist in ADD/ADHD what is causing the problem, they generally say they don't know. I am not aware of any other doctor besides myself who approaches these conditions from a hormonal standpoint. Simply put, I view ADD and ADHD as a matter of too little progesterone, too much insulin, and, in the case of ADHD, too much adrenaline. My philosophy is so far removed from the standard of medical practice, which calls for the use of dangerous stimulants to treat the problem, that it can create concerns for traditional practitioners. Yet, as they say, the proof is in the pudding. When I treat the symptoms of ADD and ADHD with progesterone and a diet that encourages the lowering of insulin, there are positive results.

The immediate response of one patient, a 53-year-old male, after starting on progesterone was that it made him extremely tired. As soon as he said that, I realized he was an adult with ADHD. He was a trim male, working a 12-to-14-hour day. Placing him on progesterone prevented his insulin levels from rising. It took away his hypoglycemia, so his adrenaline levels went down. I adjusted his diet, providing more carbohydrates to normalize the sugar, and also gave him thyroid. As a result, his fatigue disappeared.

I think part of the reason why ADD/ADHD is under-diagnosed is that doctors approach it as a "learning problem." My feeling is that this is not true. People with ADHD have no trouble focusing on things that interest them; however, they will not focus on anything that they have no interest in. In other words, ADHD is not a learning disorder; it is, more correctly, an interest disorder.

Interestingly, most of the patients I see in my practice are adults with unrecognized ADHD.

CHARACTERISTICS OF ADHD

The typical adult with ADHD has a history of increased physical activity as a teenager, being slim during his or her youth, never opening a book in high school or college until the night before an exam, and possibly becoming a type-A personality or workaholic. They usually have a history of being easily irritated and quick to anger, and they might have high expectations of other people. As they approach their middle years they start putting on weight around the waist. They have symptoms of hypoglycemia: sleepiness in the late afternoon or while driving or after eating. They commonly display restlessness—tapping their hands or feet during the day, and manifesting restless leg syndrome or tossing and turning at night. All of these symptoms and behaviors can be linked with the high adrenaline levels and high-insulin, low-blood-sugar syndrome of ADHD.

There often a strong family history of associated hormonal problems—a mother with breast cancer, a sister with endometriosis, a brother with bi-polar disorder, children or nephews and nieces who are hyperactive (ADHD). Other commonly associated conditions are type II diabetes and also fibromyalgia.

Please keep in mind that adrenaline is not only a hormone but also acts as a neurotransmitter in the brain. Adults with

ADHD are often extremely intelligent as well as extremely successful. I suspect that most of the CEOs of the largest companies in the world are diagnosable as having ADHD. They use their adrenaline to become workaholics—they put in 14-hour days and rise to the top of their businesses. Likewise, I suspect that many Hollywood stars have ADHD—classic examples might include Tom Cruise, Mel Gibson, and the comic actor Michael Richards, who played Kramer on *Seinfield*. Again, most professional athletes probably have ADHD—they use their adrenaline to excel in sports.

On the other end of the spectrum, I would not be surprised if most drug addicts and alcoholics would turn out to have ADHD. They turn to drugs and alcohol to deal with the anger caused by an excess of adrenaline. Similarly, a high number of people in prison might be diagnosable as having ADHD, also people with road rage and people who abuse spouses. Certainly, anger management classes would be largely attended by ADHD sufferers.

People are sometimes characterized as left- or right-brain dominant. People who are right-brain dominant tend to be creative. I suspect that if you take right-brain dominance and add adrenaline, you wind up with a creative genius. Albert Einstein, for instance, is well-known as having a classic case of ADHD (he failed a number of subjects in school). It may have been high levels of adrenaline that made the brains of Einstein and other creative geniuses such as Da Vinci and Beethoven function so brilliantly. I also wonder whether people with autism or with Tourette's syndrome could also have an overload of adrenaline in the brain. In autism, the excess adrenaline might be manifesting as sensory overload, and so the person shrinks back from the world to decrease the amount of stimulus.

It should also not be surprising that many conditions associated with adult ADHD are considered incurable by the medical community, since, in my view, the cause is hormones out of balance—an unfamiliar concept for many physicians. These conditions include: restless leg syndrome, fibromyalgia, type II diabetes, endometriosis, menstrual migraines, and asthma, to mention a few. Yet utilizing natural bio-identical hormones, altering the patient's eating habits, and helping them gain insight into their condition often lead to a "miraculous" resolution of these very problems.

A WIDESPREAD PHENOMENON

My point is that the medical system has failed to appreciate the influence of hormones on our behavior and how they affect us clinically. I suspect there are well over 200 million adults nationwide with unrecognized ADHD. Obviously, this is rather a bold statement. But consider the people you interact with on a daily basis—those who are quick to anger, the people with nervous energy, those who are restless at night, who tap their hands or legs, who have cold hands when you shake hands with them (due to vasoconstriction of blood vessels caused by high adrenaline levels), who drink too much or use drugs. Look at the millions of women with estrogen-dominant conditions—menstrual cramps, migraines, fibroids, endometriosis—all related to low progesterone levels. How many of these women are hypoglycemic from increased insulin and put out adrenaline to bring their sugar levels up so the brain can function?

Since hormone patterns are genetically inherited, people with ADHD will have at least one parent with ADHD—possibly a workaholic mother or father, who may have had a tendency toward anger and perhaps drank too much. If they have children, each child has a 50 percent chance of having ADHD. If their spouse also has ADHD (a fairly common occurrence, by the way) then their children are 100 percent likely to have ADHD. And then there are the grandchildren.

HORMONAL IMBALANCES IN CHILDREN

CHAPTER SIXTEEN

I want to begin this chapter by noting that the relationship between childhood illness and hormonal influence has to date essentially been ignored. What I have to say here is based on logic and my own clinical observations; there are no studies to fall back on.

Before we start, I want to remind the reader of a few well-established medical facts:

- Hormones control every system of the body.
- Males and females have the same hormones but their levels differ.
- Hormones are inherited from either parent.
- At different stages in life, hormone levels vary.

It is also worth mentioning that, as in adults, an imbalance of one hormone in children often leads to an imbalance of other hormones as the body tries to adjust to the deficiency.

Girls who have started their periods may experience irregular menses, severe cramps, migraines, or other symptoms. In addition, most people are aware that we have a nationwide problem with over-weight and obese children. We are also beginning to see a significant increase in attention deficit disorder (ADD) among children. This chapter discusses all three of these problems. I'll begin with ADD.

THE MISSING LINK

It is apparent to me that the over-production of a single hormone, insulin, is associated with many metabolic problems. Insulin is the number one hormone that creates fat, especially around the middle of the body. It is the number one hormone that causes type II diabetes, and, in my opinion, it is the hormone that precipitates ADD and ADHD. (See chapter 15 for the hormonal difference between the two.)

If too much insulin is creating problems, then let's go one step further: Why is the body producing excess insulin? Although the over-production of insulin in children can be due to many factors, its causes can probably be reduced to two: The first, and not necessarily the most important, is the type of food children are exposed to. Too many carbohydrates, in the form of fruit juice, soda, cereal, chips, fries, candy, cookies, and similar foods, leads to high sugar levels and subsequently to over-production of insulin, which then puts the sugar into the fat cells.

The other factor, which may be the root cause for all the problems discussed in this chapter, is a deficiency of progesterone. I consider this the missing link.

Low progesterone is almost always associated with the over-production of insulin. If a parent is low in progesterone, they can pass this trait on to their child. A mother low in progesterone will have a medical history that shows estrogen dominance—with symptoms that include cramps, PMS, breast tenderness, nausea with pregnancy, fibroids, fibrocystic disease, and migraine headaches. The father may have a history of hypoglycemia, increased fat around the middle, type II diabetes, or symptoms of ADHD.

My own mother was estrogen dominant and wound up dying of breast cancer because of it. She had thin arms and legs and a large abdomen—classic for hyperinsulinemia secondary to low progesterone. I inherited a progesterone deficiency from her. I had ADD as a child—I used to get up and walk out of class and could not focus. They didn't diagnose ADD back then; they thought I was bored. I wasn't bored—I just couldn't pay attention. I was continuously hypoglycemic—I craved sweets. I rarely studied in high school or college, except the night before exams. I could only focus on things that interested me, like early rock and roll in high school, and bridge and poker in college. (I studied 4 hours every night once I got to medical school—but I was interested in medicine.)

I have fought with my weight all my life because my body over-produces insulin. When I first went into practice, I used to nod off between 3 and 4 P.M.—sometimes while talking to patients! Oftentimes when I was driving I had to slap my face to keep my eyes open. All these symptoms disappeared after I started using natural progesterone.

THE OVER-WEIGHT CHILD

When people are young, it is often possible to get fat to almost melt off their bodies. They have not yet reached the stage where their bodies become sophisticated, efficient machines for fat-production and maintenance of fat.

Another chapter of this book (chapter 20) deals with weight control; the approach for children is similar to that for adults, but it is easier. Very often just teaching the child (and/or the parents) how to eat properly is all that's required. Instructing them on the importance of exercise—primarily to burn sugar rather than fat—is mandatory. Adjusting hormones such as progesterone and thyroid may be necessary. Eliminating unnecessary medications, when possible, is helpful.

What would be of immeasurable benefit is if parents would unite in a campaign to eliminate the candy-juice-soda machines in the schools, and work with the school dietitians and the fast-food purveyors outside the school to offer lower-carb choices for their children.

PUTTING PERIODS IN PERSPECTIVE

When girls enter puberty, if the ovaries are not producing an adequate amount of progesterone, the pituitary sends out hormones to step up the production. In many cases, the ovaries, for genetic reasons, are not capable of increasing progesterone, but the extra stimulation increases the amount of estrogen. This extra estrogen can lead to cysts on the ovaries. Ovarian cysts can produce an excess of testosterone, causing problems with acne and excessive hair growth. This is known as polycystic ovarian syndrome (PCOS)—again, most likely caused by a deficiency of progesterone. Keep in mind, the low progesterone associated with all of the above changes also causes the production of excess insulin, creating weight around the middle. At the same time, the excess estrogen is putting on fat around the hips, thighs, and buttocks.

Very often teenage girls with menstrual problems are put on birth control pills to help with cramps or acne. However, this is treating the symptoms instead of dealing with the cause of the problem.

The cause, in my opinion, is a reduced level of progesterone. The only time a female produces progesterone is during ovulation. Birth control pills prevent the ovaries from ovulating—so these girls go from low levels of progesterone to none. Keep in mind in this regard that progesterone is one of the most important hormones in the female body.

Giving the patient a natural, bio-identical progesterone cream obtainable from a compounding pharmacy (not an over-the-counter cream because it is too weak) will eliminate the cramps; it will help clear up acne and improve PCOS. It will also help with other problems if they are present, such as PMS, migraine headaches, and asthma, as well as lowering a high insulin level and helping to eliminate fat, ADD, and ADHD. The dosage I would probably recommend is progesterone cream 100 mg/¼ tsp applied twice a day to the forearm and wrist on days 7 thru 28 of the cycle.

FINAL THOUGHTS

Again, I am very aware that I am touching on controversial areas by making recommendations on treating conditions in children with natural hormones when there have been no direct studies. The major funding for medical studies comes from drug companies, and since drug companies cannot patent natural products, it is unlikely that we will see studies pertaining to natural hormones in children for a long time. Used correctly, however, natural progesterone is non-toxic.

To put the safety of natural, bio-identical progesterone into perspective, consider this: During a woman's monthly cycle, progesterone peaks at 28 ng/dl. When a woman is pregnant, this level goes up to 450 ng/dl—a significantly high level that the fetus is exposed to for about 5 ½ months and obviously has no trouble tolerating. In fact, the high levels of progesterone aid in brain development, among other things. When progesterone is applied transdermally to an adult or child, the blood level rises about 2 ng/dl—a mere fraction of what the fetus is exposed to.

I have recommended natural progesterone for a nine-year-old girl who was having monthly migraine headaches. She had already started developing breasts and was evidently estrogen dominant, like her mother. After she started taking progesterone, her migraine headaches disappeared.

In my view, children with undiagnosed hormonal problems are likely to face a multitude of lifelong difficulties.

In my view, children with undiagnosed hormonal problems are likely to face a multitude of lifelong difficulties. Children with ADD can wind up with diabetes, weight problems, and experience difficulty holding jobs. Children with ADHD often become adults with type A personalities—workaholics—and are at risk for developing bi-polar disorder. They frequently develop chemical dependencies on alcohol, cigarettes, methamphetamine, and other substances. Very often hormonal problems lead to depression in children. Children are also prone to thyroid conditions. Girls with low progesterone and high estrogen are more likely to have difficulty getting pregnant later on and are also possible candidates for miscarriages, morning sickness, postpartum depression, fibroids, endometriosis, asthma, migraine headaches, breast cancer, weight problems, and other difficulties.

The fact is that children are being exposed to toxic drugs such as anti-depressants, birth control pills, and stimulants for hyper-activity. Wouldn't it be more beneficial to treat the actual cause of their problems by replacing the hormone that is missing?

A PREVENTABLE TRAGEDY

On December 13, 2006, four-year-old Rebecca Riley died of an overdose of drugs given to her for treatment of ADHD/bi-polar disorder. Her parents were arrested on murder charges, accused of over-medicating their daughter to "keep her quiet." Her teachers, the school nurse, the principal, her social workers, even her pharmacist, all knew she was over-medicated. She was described as being like a floppy doll, unable to sit up, and she was shaking so badly she needed help to get off the bus every day.

To me, this girl's death represents a microcosm of the tragedy of ADHD. Do you blame the parents who had ADHD themselves, the doctor who prescribed these toxic medications, the pharmacist who knowingly dispensed too many drugs, her school, or the social workers? Her death might easily have been prevented if the medical profession was aware of how hormones contribute to this condition. I strongly feel that her ADHD/bi-polar disorder might have been eliminated with proper nutrition and utilizing natural bio-identical progesterone.

In 2002, there were about 2.5 million children in the United States on anti-psychotic medication alone, and millions of others on stimulants and anti-depressants. Today there are probably more. How many have wound up like Rebecca Riley or will do so in the future?

THOUGHTS ON CHOLESTEROL

CHAPTER SEVENTEEN

Elevated cholesterol is often a barometer pointing to some underlying problem in the body's metabolic system. It's an extremely complex issue that goes way beyond what I intend to cover in this book. However, I would like to address certain factors.

The liver is the main source of cholesterol, and the raw material for making cholesterol is the fat that is stored there. The primary source of this fat is excess carbohydrates that are ingested, rather than fat that is ingested. A study was done at Johns Hopkins University to determine the effect on cholesterol of eating white meat (fish and chicken) versus red meat (all other meats). The results showed that white meat and red meat *lowered* cholesterol by the same amount.

To a large extent the thyroid gland controls cholesterol metabolism. In fact, when I went to medical school they often referred to the cholesterol level as "the poor man's thyroid test." Unfortunately, many doctors fail to assess thyroid function when dealing with elevated cholesterol because the emphasis in medicine is on treating the symptom and not the cause. Giving thyroid hormone can very often lower the cholesterol level.

Most people are aware of HDL and LDL as two types of cholesterol. These are actually lipoproteins that transport cholesterol throughout the body. Both are necessary for proper health. LDL has a reputation for being "bad" because it can oxidize and cause damage to the coronary arteries. HDL is considered "good" because it prevents LDL from oxidizing: the higher the HDL level, the better. There are studies indicating that more people with low total cholesterol levels have heart attacks than those with high levels. If this is the case, then presumably the issue is not the level of cholesterol but whether or not it is being oxidized.

It is estimated that 20 percent of the American population has Syndrome X, a disease of hyperinsulinemia, or high insulin. Insulin puts sugar not only into fat cells, where it gets converted into fat, but also into the liver—where it also is converted into fat. This is the primary fuel used to manufacture cholesterol. If someone has high LDL cholesterol and also has a low HDL cholesterol and an elevated triglyceride level (the hallmarks of Syndrome X), lowering their insulin level often helps bring the total cholesterol level down.

As people get older, hormone levels go down, and most hormones are made with cholesterol. One theory says that the rise in cholesterol levels as we get older is partially a response by the body to the lowering of our hormones, that is, it is trying to provide more substrate to raise our hormones. Along these lines, one might anticipate that bio-identical hormone replacement would lead to a lowering of cholesterol.

STATIN DRUGS AND COENZYME Q-10

The largest-selling drugs in the world are Lipitor and Zocor. Other statin-type drugs that lower cholesterol by preventing cholesterol production include Pravachol, Mevacor, Lescol, Crestor, and Vytorin. All these drugs have the same side effects, which include brain damage and memory loss. Perhaps this is not surprising, given that most brain tissue is made up of cholesterol and there are special cells in the brain that produce cholesterol. I suspect that years from now, statin drugs may be implicated in an epidemic of Alzheimer's and Parkinson's disease. They can also cause damage to the liver, nerves, muscles, and the heart. The most serious side effects are irreversible kidney failure and sudden death.

One of the most powerful antioxidants for the heart is coenzyme Q-10. As people get older, the body produces decreasing amounts of this element. Because of this, there are probably no benefits to taking a statin drug after the age of 60.

Statin drugs lower coenzyme Q-10 levels, which is what produces the majority of the side effects of these medications. Obviously, if you are taking one of these drugs, I would recommend also taking coenzyme Q-10. It is available in drug stores and health food stores. My recommended dosage is at least 200 mg a day.

One wonders if the utilization of antioxidants by themselves might be of more benefit in preventing coronary artery disease than lowering cholesterol.

A FRIENDLY WARNING

Many people have heard of Vioxx, a pain medication removed from the market because of cardiac concerns. Recently a jury awarded 253 million dollars to the wife of a patient who died of a heart attack while on Vioxx. This sum was primarily punitive damages, because evidence at the trial indicated that the manufacturer had been aware of cardiac problems associated with Vioxx for many years. In point of fact, this was not secret information. The association between Vioxx and heart attacks was generally well publicized in various studies but unfortunately was not noted by the physicians, who prescribed 2.3 billion dollars worth of the drug per year. In my view, the jury was saying: we understand that drugs can cause serious side effects, and if a drug company knows that a certain segment of a population (e.g., heart patients) should not take a certain drug, then the company should let the FDA and the drug-taking population know it, too, and send out "Dear Doctor" letters.

That brings us to the medication Zocor, made by the same pharmaceutical company. Right now, it is the number one selling drug in the world. Side effects of the drug include brain damage, memory loss, nerve damage, irreversible kidney damage secondary to severe muscle damage, heart damage, and sudden death. Most, if not all, of these side effects are related to the lowering of coenzyme Q-10, an extremely potent antioxidant that the heart cannot function without. Sixteen years ago the company that manufactures Zocor received a patent for a new formulation of Zocor that includes coenzyme Q-10. When the time comes for statin-type drugs to be scrutinized more for safety, this fact may come back to haunt the manufacturers. It may represent another example of prior knowledge of potential problems and not publicizing the fact that all people taking statin drugs should probably also be taking coenzyme Q-10.

MORBID OBESITY AND ROGER P.

CHAPTER EIGHTEEN

Roger P., 47, arrived for his intake interview weighing 420 pounds. His pear-shaped body was the classic body type for someone who is pouring out excess estrogen along with too much insulin.

His hormone imbalance was accompanied by a host of other problems. He was reclusive, a drinker, and his body was in constant pain. As Roger tells his story, the reader will appreciate the extent of his struggle against obesity, which created devastating physical and emotional havoc.

I've been fat my whole life. Being the fat kid in school made me an outcast. When you're always on the outside looking in, your level of caring declines. I felt that everything and everyone was against me, and I was an angry kid.

Not only was I fat but I was weird looking, too. I carried all my weight in my hips and thighs, like a woman. I was one of those obese people who seem to be not a "he" or a "she" but an "it." I looked like two different people stuck together.

In my line of work, which is designing and building binary data systems, I'm able to work solo as a contract employee. I always chose to work from home, going in for meetings as infrequently as possible. I fashioned my career to allow for maximum reclusiveness.

I was always ashamed and embarrassed. Whenever I went out to eat I would find the darkest, most secluded corner in the restaurant to hide out in. Clothes were a problem, too. For years I wore bib overalls, the monster size. I couldn't button them all the way up on the sides.

And I lived in fear of children. Children would see me in public and pipe up with something totally humiliating. I started scheduling my visits to the market for the middle of the night just to avoid being humiliated by little kids.

In the midst of all of this humiliation, I had a strong feeling that this obesity was not my fault. I would keep going to doctors to try and get some help. Normally their response, after they'd taken my money, was to say, "Go home, kid, and quit eating so much." I would tell them, "I don't eat that much," and I didn't, I never have. You and I could eat the same exact meal and you'd be unaffected, but I'd wake up the next morning and my pants wouldn't fit. But every doctor I tried to get help from told me that although I probably didn't think I was a huge eater, in reality I was. They made me feel like a liar. Some of them gave me amphetamines.

At age 23 I started getting leg pains, and then later on I developed full body cramps. I was cramping all the time, having night sweats and weird vision problems. None of the doctors I went to had any solutions for me. These problems were variously misdiagnosed as gout, pseudo-gout, tendonitis, and a bunch of other things.

My life was miserable. I'd do my work, come home, drink a six-pack of beer and a half bottle of Tequila every night, and go to sleep and get up and do the whole thing over again. One night a friend infuriated me on the phone by telling me I was like some little old lady with her two dogs and no life. It sent me off the scale. I yelled at her. But I thought about it all night, and the next day

I realized that she had only described me as I really was.

I had heard Dr. Platt talking about weight loss on the radio. The day after the fight with my friend I went to see him. He sat me down and talked to me for over an hour. He wanted to know everything about my family history and my life. After my initial visit he put me on progesterone and DHEA and started me on the diet. Right away I started losing weight.

About three months into the program I had a real bad flare-up in my knee, hip and in between; it felt like having hot steel shoved up your leg. I tried a chiropractor and then a sports medicine specialist, but they didn't help. Finally I thought, "What the heck; I'll ask Dr. Platt about it."

I was totally shocked by his reaction. "Look, I'm your physician and I'm treating you," he said. "I want to know everything that's happening to you." I found that such a strange attitude for a doctor.

He added testosterone and thyroid to my medications, and changed the type of DHEA I was taking. That same day he diagnosed my fibromyalgia, which is the pain in my leg that had been misdiagnosed by so many doctors. About three days later I felt as though I'd come out of a fog. It's hard to describe. I had been there so long I didn't know I was there. I had an amazing change, a new clarity of thought. It was startling.

And I was pain-free for the first time in 24 years. Strange things started happening to me physically at this point. All my life I've been kind of a big, white farm-boy-looking guy without any muscle definition at all. Now I've developed all this muscle definition. I'm much stronger. I used to sleep eight or ten hours a night and then sit all day without wanting to do anything. Now I sleep about four hours a night and I'm never tired. Life is good.

I weigh 195 pounds. It's the first time I've been less than 200 pounds since I was 12 years old. My brain hasn't kept up with my

*body and my biggest challenges now are social and psychological.
I'd say socially I'm probably at a junior high school grade level
because I've never participated in society outside of work.*

*People sometimes ask me if I'm bitter about all the years when
I was looking for help and doors were being shut in my face. But
I'm not. They were blessings and gifts even though they were
painful. I'm pretty happy with who I am now.*

THE PAIN OF MORBID OBESITY

To me, Roger's case highlights the pivotal problem with the way
medicine is practiced today.

As I've said before, too many doctors don't have the time it
takes to listen to their patients any more. For years Roger went
from doctor to doctor about his weight problem, telling them
that he didn't over-eat and asking for help. But they didn't
listen to him. They dismissed him.

And they didn't observe him. They didn't look at him. It
was so obvious from the distribution of his fat that there was
something more than an eating problem going on. He had to
have a hormone problem—it was unmistakable. It's amazing
to me that so many doctors were blind to it.

When I went through medical school, we had a course
called "Physical Diagnosis," and it was fascinating. We learned
about an array of outward physical signs, many of them very
subtle, that you could observe in a patient to pick up information about what might be going on inside their bodies. It was
a kind of visual detective work. It kept you attuned to what
you were really seeing when you looked at your patient.

I wonder if they even teach this course any more. The
medical profession has become so fixated on technology that
simple first-person observation seems to have lost its value.

TWO STEPS FORWARD, ONE STEP BACK

This may sound strange, but I often feel that the development of blood tests has been a major setback in medicine. In the old days—going back 100 or 200 years—the only thing doctors had to rely on was talking to their patients and observing them. (In the really early days they didn't even have stethoscopes. They'd roll up a piece of paper and listen to people's hearts through that.) Today doctors have blood tests to fall back on, and they seem to find the statistical "hard facts" of blood tests reassuring. It seems that they would rather treat the blood test than look at the patient and find out what's actually going on. With every technological advance it seems as though doctors recede further and further from direct contact with their patients.

Roger was obviously crying out for help, and nobody would give it to him. He was just about suicidal when he came to me. Looking at him, at the way he stored fat in the abdomen and buttocks, it was obvious to me that his body produced too much insulin and estrogen. So I put him on progesterone right away. He went on the diet, and I eventually added other hormones to help him with his metabolism and muscle mass.

THE ROAD HOME

As he lost weight, Roger's anger melted away too, and that helped to mitigate his fibromyalgia. This man had been furious for practically all of his 47 years. He'd been a fat child, and we all know how cruel children are to the fat kids at school. As an adult he carried this humiliation with him, becoming a recluse and living a life of quiet desperation. The suppressed anger he felt must have been crushing.

Once he finally got help at our office, once he talked to a doctor who confirmed that he was not over-eating and he was not the cause of his own disfigurement, his gratitude knew no bounds. Today Roger will tell anyone who will listen that he'd walk through fire for me or anyone in my office.

If you saw Roger now, you would never know this man had once been morbidly obese. He looks like a normal person, and his entire life has been transformed. And it was so simple. It was just a matter of getting his hormones in balance and getting him to eat in a way that would force his body to burn fat.

THE INFORMATION IS AVAILABLE

The sad thing is that what I'm doing for people like Roger is based on information that's available to any doctor who wants to avail himself or herself of it.

The other day I saw an ad in the newspaper with the headline "An Amazing Weight Loss Discovery." The ad was for a pill that "causes the body to get rid of fat in three different ways." You wouldn't have to change anything in your lifestyle; you could still eat everything, you wouldn't have to exercise, and the fat would just come right off.

I'm sure you've seen such ads and scoffed at their disingenuousness. They all have little disclaimers way down at the bottom of the page, usually next to the before-and-after photos that are captioned "Results not typical." Well, if these aren't the typical results, then why buy the pills? They typically don't work! It says so right there in the ad!

I'm being a bit facetious here, but it's for a good reason. I'm trying to drive home the point that as a society we tolerate all kinds of ridiculous misinformation about weight loss, while real information that could actually help people goes unheeded.

It's my hope that people suffering from morbid obesity will take this book into their doctors' offices and demand the simple, inexpensive solutions to their plight that they deserve.

A HAPPY ENDING

At the time Roger, at age 47, first walked into my office, he told me he had never had a date in his life. He started on the program, lost weight, got down to a size 32 waist, eliminated his fibromyalgia, started dating, got engaged … and is now happily married.

It is truly miraculous what a little natural hormone balancing can accomplish.

WEIGHT LOSS— HOW MEDICATIONS CAN PREVENT IT

CHAPTER NINETEEN

Many of the medications commonly prescribed by doctors today affect people's ability to manage their weight. Some of these effects are publicized and some aren't. For instance, most people taking Prozac know that it causes weight gain, and they make a conscious choice to sacrifice optimum weight management in order to get an improvement in their emotional outlook.

But the lipogenic (fat-creating) effects of some other medications aren't well known. People who take these medications may be struggling with their weight, unaware they're fighting a losing battle against an unrecognized enemy. These people should at least know what they are up against.

ANTI-DEPRESSANTS

Anti-depressants are a major source of weight gain. I suspect this is the case in part because anti-depressants may elevate estrogen levels.

SSRIs (selective serotonin reuptake inhibitors) like Zoloft, Paxil, Effexor, Celexa, Lexapro, and Prozac are particularly prone to causing weight gain. Some doctors prescribe these anti-depressants to help people lose weight by elevating their serotonin levels—serotonin is the neurotransmitter in the brain that takes away cravings. People who have a weight problem only because they crave certain foods can sometimes find benefit in taking anti-depressants. But for the most part, people on anti-depressants will gain weight.

The tricyclic anti-depressants like Elavil, Desipramine, and Norpramin also cause weight gain.

A common phenomenon in our society is that people who are depressed about their weight start taking anti-depressants to help them manage their depression. But then the anti-depressants cause further weight gain, making these people feel even worse about themselves. It's a vicious cycle.

In my experience, the only anti-depressant that possibly doesn't cause weight gain is Wellbutrin.

BETA-BLOCKERS

People taking beta-blockers are almost guaranteed to gain weight. Drugs like atenolol, Lopressor, Ziac, and Inderal block adrenaline from entering the bloodstream. Adrenaline is what the body uses to stimulate the release of fat from the fat cells. If you can't get fat out of the fat cells, the muscles can't burn it.

Beta-blockers are also anti-thyroid drugs, as I mentioned in chapter 3. One of the treatments for someone with an over-active thyroid is to give them a beta-blocker to quiet the thyroid down. It prevents the conversion of T4 into T3, something we also saw in chapter 3.

Ironically, the biggest prescribers of beta-blockers are cardiologists, who give it to patients because it decreases the workload of the heart. I call this an irony because obesity is a major risk factor for heart disease. What they are prescribing to reduce the heart's work will ultimately give the heart more work—in the form of excess weight the patient will soon carry around.

Beta-blockers very quickly reach a point of diminishing returns for patients at risk for heart disease. The weight these patients gain cancels out many of the benefits the beta-blockers might offer at the outset.

ESTROGEN

Perhaps the biggest influence in the tendency to gain weight in women comes from estrogen. I say this because estrogen is one of the largest-selling drugs in the world, and it is prescribed to women throughout their lives, whether in the form of birth control pills in their youth or as part of hormone replacement therapy after menopause. Estrogen is lipogenic—it encourages the accumulation of fat—and this is true of both natural and synthetic estrogen.

Women who still have their uterus are conventionally prescribed a progestin along with any estrogen they are taking, since unopposed estrogen has been found to cause cancer of the uterus. The progestin most commonly prescribed is Provera, which helps protect the uterus from cancer. But progestins are also lipogenic and, like estrogen, produce cellulite and fat and increase the risk of breast cancer.

Women who take Depo-Provera shots for birth control are practically guaranteed to gain as much as 20 pounds of weight.

DIURETICS

Many people take diuretics for high blood pressure, and these medications can elevate blood sugar. Anything that elevates blood sugar will increase insulin production, and as I've said before, insulin is the fat-storing hormone.

ANTI-INFLAMMATORY DRUGS

Patients taking anti-inflammatory medications very often report an immediate weight gain. This increase in weight is probably a result of fluid retention.

STATIN DRUGS

Statin drugs, like Lipitor, Zocor, Pravachol, Mevacor, Lescol, Vytorin, and Crestor, can also cause weight gain. This is because they lower coenzyme Q-10 levels, preventing the conversion of T4 (thyroxine) into T3 (triiodothyronine), the active thyroid hormone. And people concerned with weight want their thyroid to be functioning as well as possible.

Interestingly, the most commonly prescribed drugs in this country all tend to cause weight gain. Could this be contributing to the epidemic of obesity in this country? Could this be why people almost always put weight back on after they struggle to lose it, and why some people cannot lose weight, no matter what they do?

PERMANENT WEIGHT LOSS

CHAPTER TWENTY

From the beginning of my clinical career, my approach to medicine has been preventive. It always made a lot more sense to me to prevent disease rather than to treat it.

As an internist, I continuously deal with patients concerned about their weight or trying to cope with obesity. This condition is clearly wreaking havoc on many levels. If my patients could manage their weight, the task of creating over-all wellness would be eased greatly. In other words, I have found that weight management fits easily into a category of preventive medicine.

From the outset I have been struck by these interesting statistics:

- 98 percent of people who lose weight gain it all back again within five years.

- Obesity is the second leading preventable cause of death (smoking is number one).

What if there was a type of cancer that had a 98 percent relapse rate after it was treated? Who would be happy with that type of success rate for a cancer? Patients would demand an alternative approach. But for the last 50 years, Americans have bought into the traditional, time-worn medical advice that "you have to diet, exercise, and watch your fat intake" in order to manage your weight. Sound familiar?

By now you should have an understanding of my point of view about weight management, including my conviction that embarking on a weight loss program entails more than determination and will power. Balancing one's hormones, eliminating certain drugs, and acquiring fundamental knowledge of certain nutritional guidelines set the stage for a successful approach to weight loss and wellness.

In this chapter I lay out the logic of how to achieve permanent weight loss.

THE DISEASE CALLED OBESITY

I feel that a major cause of our current epidemic of obesity is that most physicians have been reluctant to look at obesity as a disease and continue to see it as an eating problem. Doctors have an absolutely clear understanding that conditions like hypertension and diabetes are real diseases that cannot be managed using will power. They are not reluctant about helping their patients manage these conditions, even if it means treating them over their entire life span.

But obesity, they feel, can be treated with unsophisticated advice and without addressing the underlying cause. If it's not a disease, why look for a cause? This is like trying to treat a cancer without treating the cause of the cancer.

I prefer a more scientific method. Let's look at the traditional approaches to weight management to get an understanding of why they don't work.

WHY CUTTING CALORIES DOESN'T WORK

The problem with calorie restriction (dieting) as a weight loss strategy is that it triggers the body's survival mechanisms. When we limit our meal plans to 1,200 calories per day or less, the body gets alarmed. Is starvation in the offing? Best to start storing and locking away fat in earnest.

The body is a complex, multi-layered operating system. It has a whole arsenal of techniques for maintaining homeostasis and for ensuring survival. This is something that dieters forget. They become fixated on counting calories, assuming that a body deprived of energy will burn its own fat to survive. But they are wrong. A body deprived of energy will go after its own muscle tissue before it will burn fat. And in the meantime, it will marshal its powerful hormone system to alter the way it metabolizes food for energy.

People who lose weight on a diet are fooling themselves. They get on the scale and see that they weigh less, but they shouldn't be celebrating. They've just burned up muscle tissue—the only kind of tissue that burns fat. Now they have a body that's less efficient at burning fat. When they "finish" their diet (i.e., stop restricting calories) they will have less of the tissue needed to maintain homeostasis at a low weight.

> *Ninety-eight percent of people who lose weight gain it all back again within five years.*

This is why those who diet not only gain back all the weight they've lost, but typically put on an extra two or three pounds. Lost muscle tissue, together with the body's newly improved fat-storing mechanism, causes them to stabilize at a higher weight.

WHAT ABOUT EXERCISE?

Many people reason that if restricting calories is unrealistic, then the solution must be to exercise more. Exercise, after all, burns calories.

Or does it?

Exercise offers tremendous benefits to those who incorporate it into their lifestyle. It improves cardiovascular health, it makes people feel better, it's great for bones and muscles, it lowers insulin levels, and so on. However, as the sole approach to weight loss it's not what it's cracked up to be.

To lose one pound of fat by exercising, you must burn 3,500 calories. This is equivalent to going out and running 35 miles. The alternative would be walking on a treadmill at four miles per hour for 7 ½ hours.

In my practice I have come upon patients who were living on 800 calories a day and exercising four hours a day, and they couldn't lose an ounce. Talk about frustrated! These people obviously were in a severe starvation mode, and the body will not burn fat when it's starving.

WHAT ABOUT EATING LESS FAT?

Another timeworn piece of advice is to tell patients to cut out fat from their diets. Interestingly, fat is the only food substance that does not stimulate insulin. And insulin, as you now know, is the number one hormone that creates fat, especially around the middle.

Ever since this country got into a nonfat, fat-free thinking mode, we have had an epidemic of obesity. Foods like popcorn and pretzels, which are nonfat and low in calories, create more insulin than candy does. (However, the message here is not to eat candy.)

As reported in the Framingham Heart Study, which is the largest on-going heart study in the world, the men who ate the most saturated fat (butter, meat, eggs, etc.) weighed the least. Additionally, they had the lowest cholesterol levels and the fewest incidents of coronary artery disease. Fat is not the enemy.

Additionally, given that fat is the preferred fuel for survival, the body is not likely to burn it if a person restricts their fat intake. Even more important: nonfat foods are usually high in carbohydrates (sugar), so eating them causes insulin levels to increase.

THE LOGICAL APPROACH

So we've eliminated dieting, we've eliminated exercise, and we've eliminated eating less fat. Now what are we going to do?

Well, it all comes down to metabolism. The trick is to convert your body from a sugar-burning metabolism to a fat-burning metabolism. The way to do this is to take away sugar. The body gets sugar from carbohydrates. All carbohydrates break down into sugar. You must eliminate those particular carbohydrates that create the most sugar and/or stimulate the most insulin production.

It takes three days from the time you stop taking in sugar and certain other carbohydrates for your body to begin burning fat. It takes that long to get the sugar, or glycogen, out of the muscle tissue. Once you get rid of the glycogen, the usual source of energy, the muscles have no choice: they have to start burning fat. After that point, everything you do burns fat. Cleaning the house, walking out to the car, walking your dog—everything you do burns fat. Even while you are sleeping, you are burning fat.

You're still up against the fact that it takes 3,500 calories to lose a pound of fat, but now you are burning fat constantly.

Most people using this type of approach, depending upon how much they weigh and how active they are, are able to burn anywhere from 7,000 to 10,000 calories per week So their expected fat loss would be two to three pounds per week, or eight to twelve pounds per month.

SAYING GOOD-BYE TO INSULIN

Obviously, this type of approach is not for everybody. However, certain types of people have no other choice except to follow this plan. These are the people who:

- are not big eaters; they can't shave 3,500 calories from their meal plans in order to lose one pound of fat
- over-produce insulin
- have Syndrome X
- have low progesterone levels
- eat too much sugar.

For most people, insulin is the enemy. Insulin creates fat by taking any sugar the muscles have no need for and placing it into fat cells, where the sugar is immediately converted into fat. Then the insulin sits there preventing release of fat from the fat cells—it is a fat-storing hormone.

The bottom line for most people is that to get rid of fat they have to reduce insulin. If they want to reduce insulin, they have to take away sugar. Sugar stimulates insulin production.

SIMILAR APPROACHES

Cutting out carbs is the basic premise behind many weight loss approaches: Atkins, the South Beach Diet, Sugar Busters, the

Zone, Protein Power, the Carbohydrate Addict's Diet, the Mayo Clinic Diet, the Grapefruit Diet, the Stillman Diet are some of the better-known ones.

What used to be a low-fat world is rapidly converting into a low-carb world. Many restaurants offer low-carb menus, and fast food places have also jumped on the bandwagon.

This concept of eating low carb is not new. It has actually been around for more than 150 years. There were several successful low-carb programs in the 1800s, though they eventually died out. The idea was resurrected in the 1970s by Stillman and Atkins. Now there are low-carb proponents of all kinds.

One must be aware that no single diet plan is for everybody—there is no "one-size-fits-all" approach. For example, one diet plan allows a "reward meal" at supper (eat as many carbohydrates as you want within the space of an hour). People with hyperinsulinemia—which is perhaps the majority of people with weight problems—will not be successful on this meal plan. I had a patient for whom a half cup of split pea soup would prevent her from burning fat for seven days. For some people, one piece of bread, one carrot stick, or one yam will prevent fat-burning for three days.

Other low-carbohydrate plans give people the impression they can eat as much protein as they want. But this is misleading. The body cannot store protein. Any excess protein the body can't use or eliminate is converted into sugar for fat storage. In this situation, you can be burning fat (i.e., be in ketosis) and be storing fat at the same rate, and you will not be losing weight.

ADDITIONAL THOUGHTS ON WEIGHT LOSS

In order for the body to burn fat, you have to feed it and water it. The first requirement means that you cannot skip any meals. The body requires fuel 24 hours a day: your heart is beating, you're breathing, and there are thousands of chemical reactions occurring all of the time. When you skip breakfast, you are going without fuel for 15 hours. In response, the body will automatically store fat for the next 24 hours. So even if you are not hungry in the morning, it's probably wisest to eat.

The other requirement is water. Fifty percent of your body is water. You cannot burn fat without water. Keep an eye on the color of your urine. If it's yellow, you're dehydrated. Drink more water. Try to get your urine as clear as possible.

Alcohol does not enhance weight loss. The body likes alcohol as a fuel. It's an easy fuel to burn, and it burns at seven calories per gram, almost as much as fat. Given the choice, the body will always burn alcohol before fat. The bottom line is: if you want your body to burn fat, don't give it alcohol.

There is an old wives' tale that says if you want to lose weight, you have to give up coffee. In actuality, caffeine may stimulate insulin production, though not in everybody. People with Syndrome X (high insulin, high triglycerides, and low HDL cholesterol) traditionally have the worst problem with caffeine in terms of insulin.

To find out whether you are burning fat, you can use urine-testing strips called Ketostix, which are available in most drugstores. The end-stage of fat metabolism produces ketone bodies, and these are partially eliminated through the kidneys. If you have ketone bodies in your urine, the Ketostix will change color, indicating you are burning fat. Everyone's metabolism is different, so using Ketostix will help you to find out what you can get away with in your meal plan.

CORTISOL AND WEIGHT

Recently, there has been a lot of attention on the relationship between cortisol and fat. Listening to the advertisements on the radio and television, one could almost surmise that this is the only cause of weight problems. Let me try to put this subject in perspective. The body's main function in life is survival. Therefore, the body has become extremely efficient over the years at creating and storing fat, which it considers the most important fuel for survival.

The adrenal glands also aid in survival, since in times of extreme stress they produce hormones that help the body either fight a predator or escape. This system worked pretty well in the caveman days. After a cave person saw a saber-toothed tiger, his or her adrenal glands would produce cortisol, which would raise sugar levels to give the muscles energy for fight or flight. They would also release adrenaline to give additional energy, or to stimulate fat cells to release fat for even more energy. However, this system is set up for a stress reaction lasting about ten minutes.

In this day and age, people are subjected to stress continuously—at work, while driving, meeting deadlines, and so on. In these situations, the adrenal glands may be continuously putting out cortisol, which is continuously raising sugar levels, which is continuously raising insulin levels, which is continuously creating fat.

Whether or not cortisol is a major source of weight problems in people is not entirely clear. Suffice to say, however, that high cortisol levels do not promote weight loss.

Stress is never good for the body. The more in balance you are with your hormones and your environment, the healthier you will be. Look for areas in your life that are giving you negative energy and eliminate them. Eliminate time constraints, if you can. Say "no" to road rage.

One last point: exercise is a great way to reduce excess adrenal hormones and reduce stress, and maybe help with weight loss.

THE MAINTENANCE PHASE

In my practice, when patients reach their goal weight, they enter the second phase of the program, which is geared toward preventing fat from returning to the body. As long as a person limits the amount of carbohydrates to the amount of sugar required by muscle tissue, excess carbohydrates will not be stored as fat. In this regard, the amount of exercise a person engages in is the main determinant of weight maintenance. The body's priority is to replace any sugar that the muscles have burned with sugar—it's a survival thing. The more sugar (as glycogen) the muscles have burned, the more the carbohydrates you eat will go into muscle rather than being stored as fat.

If people do not want to exercise, they have to be more aware of their carbohydrate intake. People who produce excess insulin because of Syndrome X may require medication (e.g., metformin, also known as Glucophage) or supplements (e.g., chromium, alpha lipoic acid) to lower their insulin levels.

However, getting one's hormones back into balance and eliminating fat-creating medications are perhaps the key to successful weight maintenance. Here the most important hormones are progesterone and thyroid.

THE MISSING FACTORS

As stated earlier, statistically, 98 percent of people gain weight back after losing it, regardless of the approach they have used. This includes Weight Watchers, Jenny Craig, Lindora, Atkins, and gastric bypass. As soon as people get off any program they have followed, the weight tends to come back on. The reason is that the underlying mechanism that created the fat in the first place is still there, whether it be an over-production of insulin, an under-active thyroid, producing too much estrogen, or taking lipogenic (fat-creating) drugs.

If these factors are not addressed, your body will always be creating too much fat. Throughout this book I have introduced you to a number of my patients who had a lifetime of frustration until these factors were taken into consideration.

A SIMPLE PHILOSOPHY

My method for successful, permanent weight loss is simple. It's based on principles that have been around for a long time and have worked for many people. But it will not work unless the body's hormones are in balance.

Since hormone levels decrease as we age, the older you are, the likelier it is that your hormones may need to be adjusted. For reasons discussed throughout this book, finding a doctor who can balance your hormones successfully, using the natural hormones that involve the fewest side effects, may not be easy. A compounding pharmacy may be able to direct you to a physician who works with bio-identical hormones. And hopefully this book will provide enough information, hints, and examples to help you in your quest for proper treatment.

HUMAN GROWTH HORMONE—HGH

CHAPTER TWENTY-ONE

One hormone I have not mentioned until now is human growth hormone (HGH). It regulates how the body grows, repairs itself, and burns fat.

Interest in HGH replacement therapy has been on the increase ever since the publication of an article in the *New England Journal of Medicine* that showed HGH's rejuvenating potential. Daniel Rudman, M.D. documented the effects of six months of HGH supplementation upon 21 men aged 61 to 81 years. The results were remarkable. Every area measured showed improvement—their body fat decreased, their lean body mass increased, their skin became thicker, and their bone density increased. He said it was equivalent to undoing 10 to 20 years of aging.

Now dubbed the "fountain of youth hormone," HGH has become a star feature at anti-aging clinics around the country. Today more people are being exposed to HGH than ever before, and it may possibly be of benefit when used correctly.

QUESTIONS ARISE

However, as with any hormone, you must weigh the benefits against the risks. The primary role of HGH after age 30 is to help the body repair tissues—the growth stage is over. Giving high dosages of a hormone that can promote the growth of tissue may lead to unwanted side effects: acromegaly (enlargement of bony tissue), enlargement of the heart leading to congestive heart failure, carpal tunnel syndrome, and arthritis. As people get older, there is always the possibility of cancerous tissue sitting somewhere in their bodies. HGH could stimulate the growth of that tissue. (Note that when HGH is used in children to stimulate normal levels of growth it doubles their chances of getting childhood leukemia.) HGH is not recommended for people with diabetes.

HGH is the main hormone put out by the pituitary gland. Taking inappropriately high doses, especially over prolonged periods, can suppress the pituitary gland. It's the master gland, which can affect all other endocrine glands in the body, so this may create even more problems.

However, there are ways of elevating HGH levels without giving HGH directly. This can be done through manipulating other hormones or by giving supplements called secretogues that stimulate HGH production. This is a much less expensive approach than the usual high price tag charged by many anti-aging clinics for HGH injections.

OTHER CONCERNS

I have a lot of respect for nature. It seems to know what it's doing. When using hormones to alter the natural pattern, one must always consider the logic of it. Giving high dosages of

HGH at a time when the body no longer needs high levels may be problematic.

The same is true with estrogen replacement. A woman never stops making estrogen. It is produced, for instance, in fat cells, in skin cells, and in the adrenal glands. The high levels customarily given in hormone replacement therapy are needed only when a woman is trying to get pregnant—not a likely scenario in menopausal women. This is another situation in which the risks may far outweigh the apparent benefits.

One last thought to keep in mind: A major reason for the popularity of HGH is the high level of interest in anti-aging remedies. HGH stimulates the production of IGF-1 (insulin-like growth factor-1) in the liver. In fact, levels of IGF-1 are used to monitor HGH production. Recent studies indicate, however, that IGF-1 may actually speed up the aging process; it is considered the number two hormone to do this. Insulin, by the way, is number one.

Another concern is that high levels of IGF-1 are found in the cancerous tissues of people with breast and prostate cancer. My feeling is that the jury is still out when it comes to using HGH. It may possibly be administered safely with carefully controlled dosages and monitoring for untoward effects: edema, tingling in the fingertips, arthritic pains, and unwanted growths. However, the bottom line regarding the use of HGH is that it may be illegal to prescribe it. Congress passed a law years ago addressing the off-label use of HGH that declares it illegal to use HGH as an anti-aging drug or for other unsupported claims.

DOCTORS DON'T ALWAYS LISTEN—SHIRLEY M.'S STORY

CHAPTER TWENTY-TWO

Before she came to see me at age 50, Shirley had suffered from asthma and severe headaches for her entire adult life. Doctors were unable to help her with either problem, or with the weight gain that started in her 20s.

As I helped Shirley master her weight I was able to remove the cause of her asthma and headaches, too. I only wish she had come to me earlier. She would have been spared a hysterectomy and the removal of her gallbladder. Medical studies have shown that 90 percent of hysterectomies may not be necessary.

Shirley's story should strike a familiar note with patients who, when seeking help from the conventional medical community, feel they are being ignored and misunderstood.

For the first 21 years of my life I was healthy and skinny as a rail. I weighed around 103 pounds. Although I developed asthma as a teenager, other than that, I didn't have a lot of medical problems.

All of that changed after I had my first baby. That's when my weight began to fluctuate and I started experiencing painful headaches. I went from a size 3 to a size 13, and the headaches began affecting my ability to function. After my second pregnancy I went up to a size 18 and the headaches got even worse. I tried living on aspirin to control the pain, but it didn't work.

At the age of 45 I hit a wall with my weight. I'd always followed the Dr. Atkins diet to lose weight, but suddenly it didn't work anymore. So I tried different things. I tried eating small portions, eating low fat, low sugar, whole grains, fresh fruits and vegetables. I tried eating yogurt and popcorn and oatmeal. I thought these foods were good for me and would help me, but all they did was make me bigger.

As I got older my asthma attacks went out of control. It almost seemed as though the more weight I gained, the worse the asthma got. I started carrying my inhaler with me all of the time.

After my third baby I had gained so much weight I lost all the muscle control in my tummy. I was pear-shaped. I had skinny legs, skinny arms, and a huge stomach. My doctor at the time told me that if I tried to carry another baby I'd probably drag it on the ground so I decided not to have any more babies. I had my uterus removed. That was in 1988.

I had other medical problems at that time as well. I had to have a bladder operation—it seemed like everything was falling out of me! One day I had an attack, doubling over in pain, a very sharp pain in the whole stomach. I was taken to a doctor who diagnosed gallbladder and scheduled me for surgery. Unfortunately, after that surgery I had constant diarrhea. I also had high cholesterol. All my hormones had gone out of whack.

My doctor at the time prescribed Premarin for me and also Meridia, a diet pill for weight loss (I was up to a size 20). In an attempt to understand my failing health, I was reading a lot, and I got hold of some literature that was critical of Premarin. I shared it with this doctor. She told me it was nonsense. She said that since I did not have a uterus, I needed estrogen. She changed my Premarin to an estradiol patch, another type of estrogen.

I began waking up every morning with headaches. It got so that I dreaded going to sleep at night because I knew that when I woke up I'd have this excruciating pain. I had no energy and started experiencing hot flashes. When I discussed these symptoms with my doctor and suggested that the estradiol patch and the Meridia might not be helping me, she made me feel like a failure. It was as though it was my fault that I could not lose weight.

I was so worried about my failing health that I started talking to everyone I met looking for advice. Through a compounding pharmacist I found my way to Dr. Platt.

At our first meeting, Dr. Platt did a very thorough history on me. He wanted to know everything about my medical history, my parents' medical history, my sister, my husband, everything. He had me take a blood test on my first visit. He did a complete hormone panel and, after looking over the results, explained what was going on in my body. He told me that the food I had been eating was affecting my insulin levels. He explained what happens throughout the day when you eat those kinds of foods. He could see from my history and my blood tests that I was already making too much estrogen and certainly didn't need to take more. Dr. Platt was concerned about my daughter as well, since my family has a history of breast cancer and uterine cancer. He told me to stop taking the estradiol and the Meridia, and he put both me and my daughter on natural progesterone.

He told me that my other doctor wasn't lying to me; it's just that she was misinformed about natural hormones. He also gave me a book, Metabolic Solutions, *that reviewed all the things that he told me about. He said I was to commit myself to a program that he would design for me. He said I would lose my weight, have more energy, and my headaches and hot flashes would probably go away too.*

A nutritional counselor in his office set a goal weight for me and designed a meal plan that included shopping tips and foods to buy. He told me to wean myself off sugar and caffeine. The day after I saw the counselor I was at work and I started to get weaker and sicker until by evening I thought I might be dying. I called the counselor, who had Dr. Platt call me back immediately. Dr. Platt reassured me that it was just my body going through a detoxification process from sugar and caffeine. He said I'd be a lot better the next day, and sure enough, he was right.

I continue to go into Dr. Platt's office once a week. When I go in, they check my blood pressure and my urine to see how much fat I am burning. They weigh me, and I get a B12 shot.

It's been easy to stay on the diet and I've lost 60 pounds. Today I don't wake up with headaches any more—a miracle! My diarrhea's gone, no headaches, no asthma, and I have energy now. People tell me all the time that I look slimmer.

I really believe that the natural hormones have helped me the most. I'm able to control my eating now because I understand when and why I get hungry. Candy and caffeine just don't seem important to me anymore. I'm also not scared of getting out of control when I get to my goal weight. I used to be afraid of reaching my goal weight, thinking I would just gain it all back and then some, just like before. I now rely on the nutritional counselors at Dr. Platt's office because they always have good advice for me. They remind me that I'm going to be introducing carbohydrates one at a time, slowly, and that they will monitor the effects on me. I haven't reached my goal weight yet, but I already feel successful.

CHILDBIRTH AND HEADACHES

Shirley's headaches began after she gave birth to her first child. That's because pregnancy and birth cause vast hormonal shifts in some women. Hormones affect every aspect of pregnancy. The most obvious example is women with low progesterone and high estrogen suffering from morning sickness and miscarriages.

During the second trimester, the placenta begins producing copious quantities of progesterone. Progesterone is the feel-good hormone, and that's why we have the cliché of the "radiant" expectant mother as she nears childbirth. However, after a woman delivers, her progesterone level suddenly plummets. At this point the cliché reverses itself: postpartum depression is a common occurrence. In Shirley's case, her normally low progesterone levels sank even further after she gave birth, bringing on the headaches.

She'd already had symptoms of asthma as a result of her low progesterone, and naturally those symptoms got worse after the birth of her child. Shirley reports feeling that her asthma got worse as her weight increased. This is not surprising, since the most likely cause of her asthma was a high estrogen level associated with low progesterone. The more fat cells a person has, usually the higher their estrogen levels. This, by the way, could be the reason for the higher incidence of breast cancer in obese women.

Shirley's feeling that it was harder and harder to control her weight through dieting as she aged is something many people can identify with. People in their 40s often become alarmed at how stubbornly fat clings to their bodies. Throughout their teens, 20s, and 30s, they were able to force themselves to shed a few pounds when they got desperate enough, but now nothing seems to work.

In Shirley's case, this was doubly true because she was over-producing insulin. Anyone who responds well to a high-protein diet is over-producing insulin. The most common reason why people over-produce insulin is that they are not producing enough progesterone, and as we get older progesterone levels decrease. This means that in middle age our bodies will produce more insulin. And insulin, as I've said again and again, is the fat-storing hormone.

SIGNS OF ESTROGEN DOMINANCE

Shirley's medical profile told me in many different ways that she was suffering from estrogen dominance. Very often, trouble with one's gallbladder is a complication of estrogen dominance. The menstrual migraines were caused by estrogen. Her pear-shaped body type is the classic body type for someone over-producing estrogen.

MERIDIA FOR WEIGHT LOSS
— A FOOL'S ERRAND

Shirley was prescribed Meridia to help her lose weight. This was an error. Meridia is, in most cases, completely ineffective for significant weight loss.

Meridia is a combination of an SSRI (selective serotonin reuptake inhibitor) and an NRI (norepinephrine reuptake inhibitor). It was originally developed as an anti-depressant. When Phen/Fen was taken off the market, the manufacturers of Meridia decided to promote it for weight loss because Meridia affects the same neurotransmitters that Phen/Fen did.

When the manufacturers of Meridia initially tried to get the drug approved by the FDA, it was rejected. It caused too many problems with elevated blood pressure. So they cut the dosage in half to reduce the blood pressure problem. Needless to say, Meridia's effectiveness for weight loss went down as well.

The whole approach to weight loss in conventional

medicine has been predicated on the theory that people eat too much and that's why they have a weight problem. The medical community, in my view, has been remiss in not addressing the true factors that cause weight gain.

Meridia might be of some benefit in maintaining weight loss because it can reduce severe cravings for food. However, it does not address getting rid of fat. The great majority of over-weight people have hormone problems: primarily, too much insulin, too much estrogen, and an under-active thyroid. They cannot start burning fat until their hormones have been adjusted.

PREMARIN/PROVERA — THE UNQUESTIONED PROTOCOL

Shirley confesses that when she challenged her doctor about prescribing Premarin, she was chided for doing so. This is very common. Estrogen is the one hormone gynecologists know about and believe in, and Premarin is a formulation they're very familiar with. It's common for gynecologists to look askance at any question concerning Premarin's effectiveness.

Premarin is one of the largest-selling estrogen preparations in the world—although sales dropped to half what they had been after release of the Women's Health Initiative in 2002. This is a drop of 10 million prescriptions per year—resulting in a decrease of 14,000 cases of breast cancer per year. At the turn of the last century, the incidence of breast cancer was about one case per 94 women; the present rate is about one in every seven or eight women. This increase may be attributable to our friend estrogen.

I have had women patients come back to me and report that their doctors forbade them to take the natural bio-identical progesterone I had prescribed and sternly insisted that they continue their estrogen replacement therapy. I've heard of doctors who told women to throw their progesterone cream in the trash.

Some time ago, I had a 59-year-old woman in my office. When she was 52 she was started on Premarin and Provera. By age 58 she had contracted breast cancer and they removed both breasts. The doctors then prescribed what is called an Estring, which is a high dose of estradiol (one of the three types of estrogen) inserted vaginally. So now she had estrogen sitting right next to her uterus. Keep in mind that estrogen is the only known cause of cancer of the uterus.

> *Doctors have to go back to listening to patients.*
> *There is no substitute for it.*

This woman's sister had had cancer of the uterus, which indicates that the woman was genetically predisposed to contracting uterine cancer. Sitting there in my office with her husband right next to her, she told me that she was due to have another Estring put in, as she has to have a new one inserted every two months. She was arguing with me about how she wanted to have that Estring put back in. I asked, "Why would you want to do that?" She replied that two gynecologists had told her that it's safe.

I was dumbfounded. "You've already donated both breasts; you want to give them your uterus as well?" Her husband couldn't believe her, either. But women have been brainwashed regarding the purported benefits of estrogen.

Provera is just as harmful as estrogen. It is a synthetic progestin, and although its chemical name is medroxyprogesterone, it has no relationship to natural bio-identical progesterone. Many doctors unfortunately think Provera is the same as progesterone. Provera is damaging to blood vessels (like estrogen), is lipogenic (it creates fat just like estrogen), and also increases a woman's chance of getting breast cancer (just like estrogen). However, in most cases it does prevent uterine cancer, which is why it is given to women taking Premarin who still have a uterus.

HORMONE RECEPTOR SITES

Hormones travel through the bloodstream in minute quantities. When they reach a receptor site that fits them, they attach to it and are able to influence the cell they have attached to. One woman who is estrogen dominant (i.e., has high estrogen and low progesterone) may have completely different symptoms from another woman who is also estrogen dominant because their receptor sites differ.

Shirley developed asthma in her teenage years, a common problem induced by estrogen not only in women but in men as well. Her asthma got worse as she got older, for several reasons. Her progesterone levels were falling, and very likely her estrogen levels were going up as she got fatter. Fat cells produce estrogen. As we have already seen, this may explain, at least in part, why obese women are more prone to breast cancer than women of normal weight.

Shirley apparently also has estrogen receptor sites in her temporal arteries, which explains her migraine headaches. Many women have excess receptor sites in the uterus and breasts, prompting severe menstrual cramps and breast tenderness during their periods. Later on, this intense stimulation leads to uterine fibroids or endometriosis, fibrocystic disease of the breasts or ovaries, and can result in uterine, ovarian, or breast cancer. None of these conditions occur when the body has enough natural progesterone to protect these organs.

Shirley describes herself as having a pear-shaped figure. This is the case when the body is producing an over-abundance of two different hormones—insulin and estrogen. Insulin puts fat on around the waist, and estrogen puts fat on around the hips, buttocks, and thighs. This is true for both men and women. People with excesses of insulin and estrogen often have gallbladder problems as well.

TAKING THE TIME TO LISTEN

To this day Shirley remains angry about how she was treated by the medical establishment. This is not unusual. Many patients tell me horror stories about being treated in a patronizing manner and not listened to. Until there is a change in doctors' attitudes, patients will continue to be misdiagnosed, with their symptoms being addressed instead of the underlying cause. Doctors have to go back to listening to patients. There is no substitute for it.

Shirley was obviously hormonally challenged. A basic familiarity with natural bio-identical hormones on the part of her earlier doctors would have allowed her to eliminate her asthma, which would have delighted her, to eliminate her headaches, which would have amazed her, and to get rid of her fat, which would have pleased her.

Needless to say, for Shirley, using bio-identical hormones was nothing short of miraculous.

BATTLING THE MEDICAL ESTABLISHMENT— MARGARET O.'S STORY

CHAPTER TWENTY-THREE

Margaret O. is a well-educated woman, an accomplished musician and a teacher. She came to me at the age of 67, having spent the previous 37 years seeking the solution to a serious weight problem. She had been a size 22 for most of her adult life, even though she was physically active and ate healthy foods in reasonable quantities. But she had a hormonal profile that made her body store fat.

I want you to hear her story because I see so many women like her: well-educated, inquisitive, avid readers who study health and medicine in an attempt to understand their own bodies. Their weight problem isn't their fault, but the medical establishment thwarts their honest efforts to break through their difficulties.

When I started gaining weight in my 30s I wanted to find out why. I wasn't eating any more than I had been before the weight gain, and my level of physical activity was the same. Instinctively I knew some other variable was at work here. At first I went to the doctors at Kaiser Hospital, where I have my medical plan. I thought they could help me.

They did a series of tests on me and declared that I had an under-active thyroid. That made sense to me and I was hopeful that with thyroid medication my metabolism could be ratcheted up and my weight would start to go down. They prescribed the thyroid hormone Synthroid. I took it, but nothing happened.

So I went back to Kaiser and told them I was still gaining weight. They gave me the same tests over again, and they gave me another prescription for Synthroid. It seems this was the only thing they knew. When I went back a third time and told them I wasn't getting any results, they just looked at me strangely and told me to eat less.

From this experience I learned to harbor a healthy skepticism about the medical profession. Today I seek my own conclusions and I don't take things at face value any more. Being an educated person, I began reading everything I could about how the body metabolizes food. Meanwhile, I tried every diet that came down the pike. I tried Optifast, Shaklee, and many other diets. I would lose weight on each of these, but I never lost fat—always muscle. I would look at myself in the mirror after each of these diets and see flesh just hanging on me. The diets were hard to stay on, and they made me weak. I remember one time about six years ago: I was on a vacation in Hawaii after completing a diet that consisted of eating nothing but protein drinks four times a day. There I was, hiking along this trail, and when our group came to a small fissure on the trail everyone leaped across it. But I couldn't get my body to do it. I was that weak. Every time I came off one of those diets, I gained back more than I had weighed before. This went on for my entire adulthood. I got up to 240 pounds, and I am only 5'1" tall. It became hard to move around and hard to go shopping. Clothes were a problem, so I either sewed or bought them from the Nordstrom catalog. I was a size 22. One doesn't find beautiful clothing in those sizes. The simple act of getting up from a chair or a sofa was hard for me. So was going to a restaurant and sitting in a booth. I never knew whether I could fit into the booth.

I went on like this for 37 years, seeking answers, talking to people, trying diets, and joining support groups. Many times I got tired of searching and just let myself go. But even when I'd given up and gotten sloppy again, there was always part of my mind sort of passively available, listening, waiting to find out about something that might make permanent weight loss possible.

My first break came during menopause, when I read Dr. John R. Lee's What Your Doctor May Not Tell You about Menopause. This book had a lot of inside-track information about hormone replacement therapy. It gave me information about hormones that I had been seeking all my life. Dr. Lee was the first doctor to come out saying that Premarin and all the synthetic estrogen hormones being given to women at menopause were actually hurting them. He talked about how estrogen made the body store fat. I thought: At last! A clue! I began to believe that I had a hormone problem, one that went beyond my under-active thyroid.

But I needed more specific information, and I needed a doctor who could help me balance my hormones. I went to the endocrinologists at Kaiser, but that was a lost cause. They wanted to get me on Premarin as fast as they could! They are part of that medical establishment Dr. Lee writes about that is brainwashed about Premarin. They certainly were not about to help me.

I knew I needed to find an endocrinologist outside the Kaiser system who agreed with Dr. Lee's ideas and was ready to buck the whole system regarding Premarin. But where do you find someone like that? My entire life's experience had taught me that doctors were, for the most part, like Stepford wives; they were cheerleaders for a system that reduced reality to a few simple clichés. I was also leery of exposing myself to more insults from doctors. Whenever I would go in for these consultations about my weight, I could see exactly what these doctors were thinking. Whether they said it or *not, they gave me the feeling that they thought I was some kind of binge eater looking for a shortcut or a miracle.*

I started feeling trapped; I had the same discouraged, sort of Kafkaesque sensation like I'd gotten back in my 30s.

But then, over New Year's, my husband and I were at our condo in the desert and I saw Dr. Platt on television. Everything he said made so much sense that I made an appointment to see him!

I brought my Kaiser folder to Dr. Platt, and he did a battery of hormone tests. I found him easy to talk to. He also had me consult with one of his nutritionists. At first I was cynical about talking to another nutritionist. I have been through a lot of nutrition classes sponsored by Kaiser. That's another insulting thing they do when you are looking for help with weight loss: they make you take these classes. I've been through umpteen nutrition classes and cholesterol classes and so forth. You name it and Kaiser wants to put you through it.

Dr. Platt's team is welcoming. They really have knowledge that helps you and a way of sharing it that I understood.

Dr. Platt told me that when I lost weight my cholesterol would go down. My cholesterol was 293 when I went in there. Kaiser had wanted me to take Zocor for my high cholesterol, which is one of about three or four statin drugs on the market. But I said no. Dr. Platt and I are working on my cholesterol with niacin and thyroid. Within the first two months of starting with Dr. Platt, my cholesterol dropped 50 points.

When the hormone tests came back, Dr. Platt and I sat down and went over them. My low thyroid was still there, and Dr. Platt adjusted my thyroid, giving me T3 in addition to T4. He explained to me why the Synthroid by itself wasn't helping me. It made me angry to think I had been faithfully taking this stuff for 20 years and it had been doing nothing for me.

As I lost weight I gained energy. It became easier to do just about anything. So far I've lost 38 pounds. I weigh 202 now. But

I'm wearing a size 16 and there's no flab! I used to feel impaired, but I'm not impaired anymore. I have no problems getting up off of the sofa or in and out of a restaurant booth.

I've always been an active person even when it was a struggle to move around. I still work in a gift shop every day, sing in a choir, volunteer at my Temple, teach piano privately at home, and cook with my husband every night. My ideal weight is 141. I am confident I will get there.

NEAR MISSES

Over the years I've seen a lot of patients like Margaret—very smart people who try to approach their weight problems intelligently but still can't lose weight. I find their situations especially poignant. With all of their reading and detective work, they're nonetheless thwarted by our popular culture of dieting and our uninformed medical system. Margaret made some good inroads, but she just didn't take the right path to get to where she wanted to go. She had read Dr. Lee and understood the value of natural progesterone. Unfortunately, the type of progesterone he promotes is not in a high enough strength. He recommends the over-the-counter type of progesterone, which is 20 milligrams, and a woman generally needs about 200 milligrams a day.

Margaret also suspected that she had a thyroid problem, and her doctors determined that it was true. But they placed her on the wrong thyroid medication. This is extremely common, as you've already seen with Brenda J. and Rhonda Y. She was given the T4-only hormone Synthroid when she also needed T3. That's the most common error made by conventional doctors when treating over-weight people with under-active thyroid glands. They don't realize that people can have normal levels of T4 and still be hypothyroid. Few doctors look at a patient's T3 levels, T3 being the active hormone that regulates metabolism. The logical question here is: Why don't doctors start looking at T3 levels so they can cover all the bases for their patients suffering from hypothyroidism?

YO-YO DIETING AND WEIGHT LOSS

Margaret is the type of person who has the most difficult time losing weight. Her long history of repeated diets had turned her body into an extremely efficient, sophisticated fat-storing machine.

The body does not know about weight loss—it only understands the threat of starvation. Its main concern is survival. When insufficient quantities of fuel are consumed, it naturally thinks it may be facing starvation, so it begins to create and store fat in a highly efficient manner.

This is an important point that bears repeating. People interested in losing weight need to understand how their body operates. The body likes fat. It likes to create it and hold onto it and does not like to burn it.

When people go on starvation weight loss programs, most of the weight loss that occurs is muscle loss—the body does not want to burn fat when it is starving. Muscle weighs at least three times as much as fat, so people lose weight rapidly, which makes them happy. This happiness, unfortunately, is short-lived because there is a rapid regaining. Less muscle tissue means less room for carbohydrate (sugar) storage (as glycogen), so any excess is apt to be stored in the fat cells. And less muscle means less fat is burned, since muscle is the fat-burning tissue of the body.

Added to this, the body becomes even more efficient at storing fat. The bottom line is: cutting calories is probably not the best weight loss approach for long-term weight management.

Fat is a very efficient fuel—it burns at nine calories per gram—and the body wisely reserves its most efficient fuel for last. A good example of this is Karen Carpenter, the singer who died of anorexia nervosa. This was a woman who placed her body in a continuous state of starvation. When they did her autopsy, they discovered she had almost no heart muscle. Her body had eaten its most vital organ rather than give up its last ounce of fat.

A MORE ENLIGHTENED APPROACH

Could anyone have been more proactive, determined, and methodical in her search for weight management than Margaret? And yet her search went on, unsuccessfully, for 37 years. That's how difficult it is to get help with obesity in this culture! It is time to change our assumptions about why people's bodies store fat. And it's time to offer patients a more enlightened and helpful approach to weight loss.

WHY WE DON'T HAVE PREVENTIVE MEDICINE IN THIS COUNTRY

Preventive medicine is almost non-existent in this country. When you talk to some doctors about preventive medicine, they think you're talking about giving flu shots. However, many people assume "preventive medicine" refers to preventing heart attacks, strokes, cancer, diabetes, and other serious conditions.

If we look at statistics, it becomes clear that over the past 60 years the incidence of these medical conditions has hardly reduced. Despite the proliferation of drugs and new medical technology, nothing much has changed.

NO PROFIT MOTIVE

Almost everything doctors learn in medical school about treating patients is based on research done by drug companies. This is why most doctors have little basic knowledge of natural hormones—drug companies cannot patent natural products. Even endocrinologists, who specialize in hormones, for the most part only feel comfortable using the synthetic hormones produced by drug companies, not natural bio-identical hormones that match the hormones produced by the body.

Along these same lines, doctors learn little preventive medicine in medical school because drug companies have no interest in preventing disease—why should they? There's no profit for drug companies in treating the root causes of heart attacks, strokes, diabetes, and cancer. The entire medical establishment is geared toward treatment, not prevention. For the most part, drug companies develop drugs to treat symptoms of disease. Antibiotics are the only drugs that actually address and cure the disease itself.

Even insurance companies—which have the most to gain from doctors practicing effective preventive medicine—play into this system by discounting the importance of proper screening procedures. By and large, insurance companies are loath to pay for simple screening tests, the kind that could help patients head off diseases they might be prone to developing. When a doctor or patient requests coverage for a blood test or any other study, the insurance company normally responds by asking for a diagnosis to support the doctor's reason for doing the test.

Well, if there is a diagnosis, the patient already has the disease. The whole point of screening is to prevent the disease from coming on in the first place.

There is a blood test called CA-125 that allows doctors to screen for cancer of the ovaries. This condition, found in one out of every 50 women, is 100 percent curable if diagnosed early and almost 100 percent fatal after it has spread. Insurance companies will not cover a CA-125 as a screening test but will pay for it once you have the condition.

This is especially galling in light of how eager the medical community is to place women on estrogen, a substance that places them at serious risk for cancer of the ovaries. Estrogen is still one of the largest-selling drugs in the world. You would think a simple, inexpensive test for cancer of the ovaries would be standard in a society that prescribes estrogen with such regularity. However, for reasons I cannot decipher, insurance companies will pay for a PSA test to screen for prostate cancer, but not for a CA-125 test.

STROKES AND HEART DISEASE

Heart attacks are the number one cause of death in both men and women. This would, of course, be a prime area to exercise preventive medicine. Yet in spite of all the measures being implemented—coronary bypass surgery, the placing of stents, angioplasty, the use of drugs to lower cholesterol, stop-smoking campaigns, dieting and exercise programs, to mention several— there has been no change in the cardiovascular mortality rate since 1950.

Is it possible that we are not addressing the major causes of cardiovascular disease?

Everybody has heard about cholesterol—the good (HDL) and the bad (LDL). Lipitor and Zocor, which reduce cholesterol levels, are now the largest-selling drugs worldwide. This fact has been greatly enhanced by the tendency to keep lowering the upper limit of "normal" for total cholesterol. When I was in medical school, a normal cholesterol level could be as high as 300. This number has been continuously lowered to the latest "normal" level of 180. Now there is talk of lowering the level to 160, which will allow doctors to place children on these drugs.

Interestingly, it has never been demonstrated convincingly that lowering cholesterol prevents coronary artery disease, and some studies indicate that more people who have heart attacks have low cholesterol rather than high cholesterol. There is, however, a much more serious risk factor that the medical community has largely ignored—the homocysteine level.

THE HIDDEN ENEMY

Homocysteine is found in everybody's bloodstream. It is a breakdown product of methionine, an amino acid. In high levels it damages blood vessels and causes them to be sticky—a risk factor for cholesterol plaques and blood clots. It predisposes a person not only to heart attacks but to strokes, Alzheimer's disease, Parkinson's disease, and osteoporosis, and it shortens the lifespan. Certainly, it's an important risk factor to screen for. However, the treatment consists of a combination of three B vitamins—folic acid, vitamin B12, and vitamin B6—along with trimethylglycine, all natural products of little benefit to drug companies.

Once again, it seems that if drug companies are not interested, doctors are rarely informed. Even if they are informed, insurance companies do not pay for the test unless there is an underlying diagnosis to support doing the test.

Another risk factor that is often not considered is called C-reactive protein (C-RP). This is a marker for inflammation in the coronary arteries—again, a situation predisposing to plaque formation and blood clots. Women with elevated C-RP levels are at significant risk of sudden death, and this element is considered a much greater risk factor than a high LDL cholesterol.

As an aside, elevations of C-RP can also be a marker for cancer of the colon and for macular degeneration, the number one cause of adult-onset blindness. Certainly, this is a screening test that should be performed, but it is rarely done. Here too, the treatment of elevated levels often incorporates the use of natural antioxidants, which are, again, substances not promoted by pharmaceutical companies.

I am a realist. As most people are aware, business runs this world. The medical system is a multi-trillion-dollar-a-year industry that sadly seems to be thriving on disease and illness, not wellness.

When studies are publicized defaming the health benefits of natural products, such as vitamin E or DHEA, it is worth considering the source. A recent study, for instance, concluded that treating elevated homocysteine levels has no clinical benefit. However, reading the actual study reveals that the researchers did not lower the levels significantly enough to have any benefit. Those studies that show no benefit, or even harm, from certain vitamins usually involve synthetic vitamins, which the body is unable to recognize.

THE MESSAGE

People are discovering that in many cases, in order to be healthy, they have to become pro-active. They have to take their health into their own hands. They cannot fully rely on a health system that is not fully committed to their being healthy.

It is my conviction that over time more and more doctors will be tuned into the use of natural hormones to prevent and heal illnesses and to screen for other preventable disorders. However, this will not happen until patients demand better approaches to their health.

BIO-IDENTICAL ISSUES

Currently there is controversy surrounding bio-identical hormones regarding their safety and efficacy. The American Medical Association (AMA) has denounced them; pharmaceutical companies want the Federal Drug Administration (FDA) to shut down compounding pharmacies.

Criticism includes the claims that bio-identical hormones are not FDA-approved and there are no long-term studies demonstrating their efficacy. Additionally, people being interviewed as experts, though they lack experience utilizing these products, contend that bio-identical hormones do not get absorbed and they provide no benefits. Wyeth, the pharmaceutical company that makes Premarin and Provera, has said that bio-identical hormones are not safe. Considering the dangers of Premarin and Provera established by the Women's Health Initiative, this is not worth commenting upon.

Let me address some of these issues.

Bio-identical hormones are manufactured by traditional pharmaceutical companies. They have a natural base, usually soy or yam, and are sent in the form of powders to compounding pharmacies, where they are then made into creams, capsules, gels, troches, and suppositories. All products manufactured by pharmaceutical companies are approved by the FDA, which dispels one of the criticisms.

Upjohn Pharmaceuticals has been manufacturing bio-identical hormone products for 70 years—to say they have not been around long enough to assess their safety is absurd.

Many studies indicating the benefits of bio-identical hormones have in fact been published, albeit not in the traditional medical journals that are basically bought and paid for by drug companies.

As for criticism that these products aren't effective, I find nothing more rewarding than hearing one of my patients state, after being introduced to bio-identical hormones, that they have never felt better. This is a statement that traditional doctors rarely hear. To know if bio-identical hormones work, I just need to listen to, and observe, my patients.

THE REAL CONTROVERSY

It is my feeling that the actual concern when it comes to hormone replacement therapy is not being addressed. The debate is mainly revolving around the type of estrogen prescribed for women during menopause—natural versus synthetic, and, if natural, urine-based versus plant-based.

However, it is my feeling the debate should be centered not on the type of estrogen a woman should receive, but on whether estrogen should be replaced at all. As mentioned throughout this book, women never stop making estrogen. They simply produce smaller amounts as they get older. Considering the risk of serious side effects associated with estrogen, if a woman in menopause is not trying to get pregnant, why try to increase her estrogen levels unnecessarily?

Please remember, the fact that a hormone is bio-identical

does not confer safety in and of itself. It still has to be used appropriately and only when necessary, just like any other medication.

WHAT IT'S ALL ABOUT

Until doctors get back to treating their patients instead of lab tests, until they start listening to patients instead of drug companies, and until they open themselves to a more logical and healthful approach to medicine, we are destined to remain on the bottom of the list of civilized countries when it comes to health care.

Not surprisingly, many physicians are becoming disenchanted with the way medicine is practiced. They recognize that they are losing control. Because of decreasing reimbursements and higher overhead costs, they are forced to see more and more patients per hour and cannot provide the time their patients may need. Insurance companies dictate to them the rules about what's covered—or more accurately, what's not covered. Drug companies besiege doctors with self-serving information, leading to more and more prescriptions for more complex medications whose side effect profiles are not clearly established. This in turn leads to drug interactions, unnecessary hospitalizations, and, not uncommonly, death.

A recent poll among primary care physicians (family practitioners and internists) indicated that 80 percent would not to go medical school again, given the choice.

Understandably, many doctors are becoming interested in a different type of practice. We are seeing a rise in practices designated as boutique, concierge-type offerings, which are able to provide a more personalized service—at a much higher cost. However, this is still a form of traditional medicine.

At the same time, more physicians are getting involved with bio-identical hormone therapy. They should understand however, that a weekend seminar in Las Vegas does not begin to cover the intricacies involved in bringing patients into hormonal balance. Nevertheless, as time goes on and physicians become more knowledgeable about bio-identical hormones and how the body functions, a whole new era in health care will be ushered in. The main force driving this revolution will be patients who simply want to feel better.

A philosopher once said
that all new ideas must go through three phases.
First, they are ridiculed.
Next, they are viciously attacked.
Years later, they are accepted as self-evident truths.
Then people say, "Oh yes, we've known this all along."

FOR MORE INFORMATION

THE INTERNATIONAL ACADEMY OF
COMPOUNDING PHARMACISTS

P.O. Box 1365, Sugar Land, TX 77487
Toll-Free Referral Line—800.927.4227
REFERRALS FOR ALL CONTINENTS
Phone—281.933.8400   Fax—281.495.0602
Website—www.iacprx.org   Email—iacpinfo@iacprx.org

PHARMACY COMPOUNDING
ACCREDITATION BOARD

P.O. Box 282, 106 S. Dodge Street, Algona, IA 50511
Phone—515.341.1250   Website—www.pcab.info

PLATT MEDICAL CENTER

72-785 Frank Sinatra Dr., Ste. B, Rancho Mirage, CA 92270
Phone—877.DR.PLATT
Website—www.drplatt.com   Email—questions@drplatt.com

INDEX